Experts and Caregivers Pr...

When the Man You Love Is Ill

"Dr. Lynn is an inspirational, compassionate voice of reason during one of the most difficult experiences that one can have in life. Dealing with the illness of a partner or any loved one is enormously stressful and this book provides the emotional support necessary to handle the challenges with grace and hope."

—RITA COSBY
Emmy Award–winning journalist, MSNBC

"As a man who knows from sad experience what a devastating impact a spouse's illness can have, I highly recommend this book as a guide for coping and caring. It is comprehensive and accessible—a true gift to people whose world is suddenly turned upside down."

—MORTON KONDRACKE
author of *Saving Milly: Love, Politics, and Parkinson's Disease*
and journalist, Fox News Channel

"As a professional caregiver, I have found Dr. Lynn's guidance invaluable in balancing the competing needs of my patients, family and self. When your own needs are left out of the equation, the caregiver can't remain giving in a full-hearted way. I know these issues from both a professional view and personal experience. I couldn't have done it without her!"

—FERN LOOS BEU, PhD

"Fearless and compassionate, with guts and gusto, Dr. Lynn shows us how to deal with one of the most challenging parts of growing older—caring for an ailing loved one."

—DEVRA DAVIS, PhD, MPH
Director of the Center for Environmental Oncology
at University of Pittsburgh Cancer Institute
and author of *When Smoke Ran Like Water*

"I believe that caretakers are truly the heroes of our society. Disabilities may not always be at the crisis level of a disease. But for a person to enjoy what life has to offer, they may need support. As baby boomers, we never thought that we'd get to this age. I feel like I traveled quickly from youth to old age. My husband, Lee Atwater, Chairman of the Republican National Committee, was sick at 39, and died at 40. I am very lucky that I had a close family network to get me through the struggles. Dr. Dorree Lynn's book shows us that everyone needs a support team to comfort us. Most importantly, never take anything for granted. Appreciate every day."

—SALLY ATWATER
Executive Director, Presidential
Committee for People with Intellectual Disabilities

"I really could have used a book like this when I went through the loss of my husband, Victor. Everyone needs to give themselves the right to grieve. If you have a loved one who is ill, what you could use is a book like Dr. Lynn's that will guide, encourage, and open up a dialogue about caregiving. I now know that I need to forgive myself for being paralyzed and not able to work following Victor's death. I walked around in a daze and had unrealistic expectations.

"I felt tremendous guilt; I thought that if only I had nagged more, I might have 'saved' him. What I tell my friends now: Never go to the doctor or hospital without a savvy advocate. Call in hospice long before you think it's indicated; they are invaluable. Tell your partner you love him each and every day. Don't wait until your husband or partner can no longer hear you."

—KAREN FAWCETT
President, www.BonjourParis.com

"One of the most challenging experiences a couple can have is when a spouse becomes seriously ill. In the past five years, my husband was diagnosed with such an illness. Since then, our lives and the lives of our children have changed dramatically—the pain and suffering, the sadness and frustrations, the new and added responsibilities on all of us—have been overwhelming! *When the Man You Love Is Ill* serves as a guiding light, providing pragmatic information on how to take care of your loved one and family, how to survive and cope, and how to empower you to take care of yourself."

—ANNIE TOTAH
community leader and philanthropist

"A timely book that offers just the kind of straightforward advice we all look for in a time of crisis. This is a book that you can carry with you and refer to time and again as new challenges arise. Everyone can benefit from Dr. Lynn's sound counsel."

—AVRUM GEURIN WEISS, PhD
co-author of *Experiential Psychotherapy* and adjunct faculty at Georgia State University, Department of Psychology

"Dr. Lynn has written a practical, no-nonsense approach to effectively navigate the uncharted waters of caring for the man you love when some of your worst fears become reality."

—EDDIE REECE, MS, LPC

"Dr. Lynn provides the sort of advice that is invaluable when caring for a loved one who has a long-term or terminal illness. She provides practical and compassionate tips on how to provide quality care, yet maintain individual balance and peace. This book would have been a tremendous help to me and my family when my father battled Parkinson's disease."

—U.S. REP. MARK UDALL (D-COLORADO)

"My husband [comedian Richard Pryor] was quoted as saying, 'God gave me this M.S. to save my life.' Richard was a fighter, and after he announced his diagnosis of multiple sclerosis, we knew that his life needed to change. We both set about to rehabilitate his health. There were many challenges: a litany of medical modalities and lifestyle changes. We met the challenges head-on and with a fierce determination to surmount them all.

"During the last years of his life and particularly the last two weeks, we would laugh and reminisce about his life and our time together. He finally came to understand the impact he had on the comedy world and also felt the love that so many had for him. It is a great challenge to care for the love of your life, especially when someone has such a life force as Richard. More difficult still is to prepare yourself for something so devastating. If Dr. Dorree Lynn's book can help even just one couple navigate the ever-changing and rigorous tides of this entire process—caring for someone you love—then every word written here has value. We all need guidance and support, and *When the Man You Love Is Ill* offers readers both honest advice and comfort."

—JENNIFER LEE PRYOR
actress

Dorree Lynn, PhD,
and Florence Isaacs

When
the *Man*
You *Love*
Is *Ill*

Doing Your Best
for Your Partner
without Losing
Yourself

Marlowe & Company
New York

WHEN THE MAN YOU LOVE IS ILL:
Doing Your Best for Your Partner without Losing Yourself

Copyright © 2007 by Dorree Lynn and Florence Isaacs

Published by
Marlowe & Company
An Imprint of Avalon Publishing Group, Incorporated
245 West 17th Street • 11th floor
New York, NY 10011

AVALON
publishing group incorporated

Library of Congress Cataloging-in-Publication Data
Lynn, Dorree.
    When the man you love is ill: doing your best for your partner without losing
yourself / by Dorree Lynn and Florence Isaacs.
        p. cm.
    ISBN 978-1-56924-285-8 (pbk.)
    1. Critically ill—Family relationships. 2. Caregivers—Family relationships. I.
Isaacs, Florence. II. Title.
R726.5.L96 2007
610—dc22

2007005331

ISBN-10: 1-56924-285-2

9 8 7 6 5 4 3 2

Designed by Pauline Neuwirth, Neuwirth & Associates Inc.

Printed in the United States of America

Contents

PART FOUR

Taking Care of You 213

Introduction

When you first get married, you naturally expect to live a life of happily ever after. Your prince is not supposed to fail you or get sick. In a committed relationship without a piece of paper, you're even less likely to anticipate that he will have health problems and that they will have an enormous impact on you. But life is unpredictable. And when the man you love falls seriously ill, your fear can feel like a knife in the heart. Suddenly everything changes. The patterns and routines that give shape and meaning to day-to-day living dissolve into chaos, testing your emotional and physical strength. You wonder how you will ever get through this ordeal.

I understand how devastated you feel. As a psychologist, I've helped couples deal with the impact of illness over thirty years of clinical practice. I know what it's like to lie awake at three a.m. with your gut in a knot, anxious about what lies ahead (not to mention taking care of your partner right now). I know what it's like to visualize to-do lists in your head and wonder if anyone will rescue you as you try to gain some semblance of control.

During those long nights when you can't sleep, you may even sob so deeply that you doubt you will ever make it to morning. My mission is to help you get through this tumultuous time, a time when you may panic or feel like you want to give up.

Clients who are struggling with a partner's illness often ask me, "How do I cope?" I tell them that the most important thing to remember is that this time of change will not last forever. It is also an opportunity, a chance to be more authentic and real—the woman you truly are—and to discover that you are stronger and more capable than you realize. If you can focus on that possibility, even though anxiety may be a constant companion right now, you will be amazed at what you can accomplish.

That does not mean you have the power to change your mate's diagnosis or cure his illness. You can't make his injuries disappear or restore his impairments; these feats are beyond your control. Nor does it mean you must be a perfect, ministering angel to a spouse. Yet you can achieve something very important. You can learn to deal more effectively with whatever has happened and help him get through it. You can be his coach and cheerleader and give him the practical and emotional support he needs, even though you may feel like you're falling apart.

To achieve this goal, you may have to change your concept of what it means to be a loving partner. Women tend to believe they have to do it all. The truth is, if you're worn out or ill, both your patience and stamina suffer. You cannot give your man the support he needs unless you value your own physical and emotional needs at the same time. To do your best for him, you must also nurture yourself.

When you are taking care of an ill spouse, part of the challenge is finding help and hope without ever losing sight of reality. Too often, people go to the bottom line, thinking, "He will never be well again." "Our life is over." "He's going to die." Perhaps in some cases, death is indeed imminent, but maybe there's also a great deal of life to live before that happens. "This trial will never end," you may think to yourself. In fact, nothing lasts forever. Emergencies do end. That's part of their definition: they have limitations and evolve into something else where adjustment is possible.

In the process of finding your way through your own situation, you're going to have to deal with the complexities of his illness, the tasks that fall on you, and all the emotions stirred inside. Some feelings may stop you from reaching out and using available assistance. Yet asking for help is a necessity. I will steer you to resources for your needs and circumstances. There are not enough of them, and the demand for scarce resources will increase as the majority of Americans pass age fifty, putting them at increasing risk for heart disease, cancer, diabetes, and other major health problems. However, because of their pride or lack of knowledge, too many people fail to take advantage of what *is* available—often very close to home.

Getting through this difficult time is a profound and individual experience. Although you ultimately navigate the shoals in your own personal way, you're also going to find you have much in common with others who struggle through a partner's illness. There are all kinds of women. Some are compassionate and nurturing, others independent. There are confident women and insecure women, working women and full-time homemakers. There are Harvard PhDs and high school graduates, CEOs and secretaries. There are wealthy women and those who scrape by. You may not read the same magazines or travel in the same circles or shop in the same stores, but you all share pain and daunting challenges. Whoever you are, you have the ability to do your best for your man.

When you're running on empty and feeling lost, you can turn to this book for gentle guidance on how to cope. I'll help you to become more aware and share with you the coping strategies that have worked for many couples I've treated. Much in our lives is accidental—powerful events happen that you simply can't control. But I've seen wives and partners emerge stronger than they thought possible, and better than ever, even in the worst situations. You can, too. And along the way, you can forge a deeper, more meaningful relationship with the man you love.

PART ONE

An Unplanned Education

Caring for an Ill Husband or Partner

He's Sick—
and You're in Charge

It started on the way to Wal-Mart. As Laura added last-minute items to her grocery list, suddenly her husband, Ralph, turned in the driver's seat and announced, "I don't feel very well." He was in a cold sweat. After reaching the mall parking lot, Ralph sat in the car while Laura shopped. When she returned with a full cart, she thought he looked worse. "You'd better see the doctor. Maybe you have the flu," she told him. That afternoon he called for an appointment. The next morning, as Ralph lay on the examining table, he had a major heart attack.

"For better or for worse, for richer, for poorer, in sickness and in health." Like most of us, Laura had heard the vows on her wedding day and repeated them, but she automatically assumed they would be tested on other people. She never dreamed that instantly the words would take on new meaning or that her life would change forever. And you probably never expected that your own partner would fall seriously ill, either. You never thought you'd be charged with his care for weeks or months, or even years.

His illness might have appeared suddenly, a thunderbolt from the blue. Perhaps he crossed the street at lunch hour, minding his own business, when a car swerved and hit him. His injuries are severe. Or maybe all he did was get a routine checkup after changing his health insurance. It never occurred to either of you that tests would reveal prostate cancer.

For my coauthor, Florence, catastrophe struck on a sunny Saturday in April. Her husband developed a cough and complained of a painful sore throat. Within days, his condition drastically worsened. What had seemed at first like an ordinary cold turned out to be a rare, life-threatening infection that put him in intensive care, hooked up to a ventilator. He was hospitalized for two months.

Other illnesses unfold differently and may invade your life gradually over a long period of time. Your mate develops a chronic disease, such as diabetes, heart disease, emphysema, or multiple sclerosis. Symptoms may come and go; there may be flare-ups and remissions. Or his illness may steadily worsen, and health issues may multiply.

When a condition progresses slowly or remains stable for a time, you may find yourself reassuring others—and even convincing yourself—that everything is fine. Yet below the surface lurk anxiety and a shaken sense of security. Whatever it is he's got, deep down you know it is not just a cold. Complications may ensue, and sooner or later reality sets in.

In contrast, immediate medical crises slap you in the face, as in Laura's case. You're burdened with demands and responsibilities you've never confronted before. You may be thrust into the roles of decision maker, manager, and nurturer, whether you're good at them or not, whether you like it or not. Whether you have young children, as Laura did, or your children are grown, as Florence's were, you may find yourself feeling overwhelmed, vulnerable, and very much alone—an unfamiliar state.

Whatever the circumstances when your own mate fell seriously ill, you're likely facing a formidable challenge: to give him what he needs even though your life feels as if it will never be the same. Chances are, it never will. But whether the tasks ahead are great or small, temporary or long term, how you come through the experience is partially up to you. As difficult as it may be, I assure you it is possible to get through it—while preserving your own health and well-being. Though the road may be bumpy, if you ask and seek, there is usually help available.

WHY DOES TAKING CARE OF YOUR PARTNER SEEM SO DIFFICULT?

"THE TOUGHEST PART was the three weeks he spent in the hospital and I stayed overnight. It completely disrupted our lives. I took my laptop so I could work there," says Karen, whose husband had brain surgery.

Taking care of an ill mate has never been simple. Today, however, a number of changes in our society make the task more demanding and complex than ever before. The majority of us wear so many hats that it's easy to lose our heads. For example, you may work full or part time while juggling child care and all of its demands—plus obligations to elderly parents. Add your mate's illness on top of that, and you're forced to cope with new daily frustrations: complicated insurance systems, pharmacy mix-ups, health care and hospital bureaucracies. No wonder you feel completely exhausted! And when that happens, you probably put yourself last.

TRADITIONAL SUPPORTS HAVE DISAPPEARED

ONCE UPON A time, people lived together in small communities. Whether the community was your town, or a few city blocks that formed your neighborhood, you had a network of others at your disposal who automatically pitched in to help in a crisis. If your house burned down, relatives and neighbors rushed over to rebuild it. When your husband fell ill, the same people delivered food to your doorstep and were there to spell you if you needed a break. You were taken care of. You had help to do what you had to do, and the community created a sense of security.

Today, for many, that scenario has all but vanished. Extended family often lives far away. According to the U.S. Census Bureau, one-sixth of all Americans move each year. If your husband is diagnosed with colon cancer after you've relocated for a new job, you haven't yet had a chance to build community and don't have instant help. Often, it's the Internet, not the phone, that connects you to friends. Resources are more diverse and no longer next door. Yet they do exist, and once you identify and harness them, they can work. Doing everything yourself has been the American way, but in this case it can be destructive to both you and your partner. One of my goals is to help guide you through the maze of support available.

THE AGE OF CHRONIC DISEASES

IN AN ERA where life expectancy is at an all-time high, medical advances have transformed killer diseases into conditions we can manage. Today, 90 million of us have one or more chronic conditions, such as arthritis, asthma, and diabetes. Many patients survive diseases that used to be fatal, and in many cases they are able to function at work and elsewhere in their lives. Your mate may be one of the millions of cancer or heart attack survivors, or a stroke survivor who has regained some or all function.

Not everyone is so fortunate, however. Even if your mate is functioning again, once the two of you have experienced such a "hit," you may never again feel totally safe. You may worry for the rest of his life about the possibility of recurrence or the increased risk for another, separate bout. You live just a little differently than before, aware that life can throw another curve ball at any time. You've entered the world that is now called "the new normal." After crises have passed, it's like living on permanent high alert, and it's difficult to endure. Yet it can be done without affecting the parts of your life that bring meaning and pleasure.

WHAT YOU CAN DO

SUCH SEISMIC SHIFTS can make taking care of your partner extraordinarily stressful, and you can't do it alone. The task is to find help and take what you need. You have your own way of doing things and your own individual circumstances. There is no "one size fits all" formula.

You can also learn to ask the right questions—not "Why is this happening to me?" but "How can I handle this most effectively?" The chapters ahead will help you to:

Map out what needs to be done in your situation.

Is it an emergency or crisis? Is he undergoing extensive treatment or recuperating from surgery? Does he suffer from a chronic disease? What will be required for you to do your best for him varies, depending on the illness, its course, the stage, whether recovery is expected, and whether he will be able to return to a relatively normal life. It also depends on whether you're involved in "caregiving lite" or heavy-duty tasks, taking care of him intermittently or on a daily basis, and whether the illness is temporary or long term. The to-do list is different for recovery from a successful heart bypass than for a stroke that dramatically curtails his life. Be assured that no matter how difficult the situation, there are often options and choices that can ease your way.

Understand the male patient psyche.

There are reasons why he won't call the doctor or take pre-scribed medication, why he grouses at you or obsesses over his condition. It's a lot easier to deal with his confusing or frustrat-ing behavior when you understand what's happening from his perspective. You're also more likely to remain loving and patient, essential ingredients for doing your best for him.

Handle your own uncomfortable reactions.

"How can I stand it?" "How *dare* he get sick?" "Get me out of here. I want to run away." "I can't bear what may happen next." "I'm drowning." Depending on the nature and severity of his illness, you may experience any or all of these responses. Or you may not feel or think at all. Instead, you may freeze and stop functioning or simply go on autopilot. You may assume you're the only one who feels this way, but you are not. You can learn ways to stay positive and productive, and to channel feelings of panic or depression into constructive behavior.

Deal with losses.

When your partner is sick, both psychological and material losses can be life changing, depending on the condition and its course. He may no longer be the man he was. The everyday things bothered Jeri: "I have to carry *his* packages and stow *his* suitcase in the overhead bin on the plane." Your lifestyle, social life, and sex life may change. It is hard to acknowledge what is gone, but it's only when you do that you can begin to reconstruct a meaningful new life.

To be sure, you'll have to make compromises. You may have to accept limits. But facing the challenges of your mate's illness can also become a transformational experience, an opportunity to discover the meaning of deeper love and commitment.

Acquire or improve caregiving skills.

Because hospital stays have grown shorter and home care has increased, you may be asked to perform tasks that used to be handled by medical professionals. Such demands on you can add more stress to an already scary experience. Few of us are born nurses or doctors. Yet fear is trumped by necessity. You may find you can learn almost anything when you must. And if you can't, there's the option of turning to other resources.

Part of your responsibilities involves learning all you can about your partner's condition so that you can be an effective advocate for him. Sometimes you have to stretch yourself to ask the most embarrassing, frightening, and important questions. When so much is at stake, it is possible to move beyond your own comfort zone to do so.

Monitor your relationship.

Your mate's illness can have a tremendous impact on your relationship as a couple, and may raise questions and issues people rarely talk about, including:

- Do I fall apart—or rise to the challenge?
- Should I stay—or should I go?
- Is there sex after prostate cancer, heart disease, etc.—and what do I do if there isn't?
- What happens to intimacy? Will our relationship ever feel the way it used to?

If you are recently remarried or just beginning a committed relationship, you may feel particularly ambivalent about devoting yourself to your man's care. A shorter-term relationship leaves you less prepared to deal with monumental events, and you may not know whether to buckle down or run. These are very human conflicts. On the other hand, the longer you've been together, the likelier you are to assume your new role without reservation. The threads of life's experiences—the births, deaths, weddings, joys, and setbacks—have already been woven into the fabric of your relationship. You know the dance of life.

Nevertheless, there are issues that can distance the two of you. I'm going to help you recognize threats to your relationship and share strategies that bring you closer together. Nurturing your connection with each other can bring joy and satisfaction—and this emotional contact actually aids physical healing as well.

Tend to your own needs.

Unfortunately, taking care of an ill family member is associated with a decline in caregivers' own health, especially when the patient is your mate. If unchecked, the stresses created by the unique male-female relationship add to the emotional and physical toll of caregiving. Results of a study of couples sixty-five and over published in the *New England Journal of Medicine* show that if your mate is hospitalized with a disabling disease, it increases *your* risk of death. Wives of men hospitalized with dementia, for example, had a 28 percent greater chance of dying within one year of their husband's hospitalization than those whose mates were not hospitalized. The more debilitating the condition, the greater the threat to caregiver health, according to research by Dr. Nicholas Christakis, professor of medical sociology at Harvard Medical School and Paul Allison, professor of sociology at the University of Pennsylvania. They speculate that stress, loss of support, or the caregiver's harmful behavior, such as drinking or poor self-care, may explain the increased risk.

To protect yourself, you may have to take a hard look at your role as a caring partner. It does not involve transforming yourself into a saint, which is an impossible goal, or destroying your sense of self or physical health. It does require a balance between sacrifice and healthy self-interest.

You play a crucial role in your partner's recovery—or in helping him adapt to his new disease or deficit. You must give yourself permission to take care of yourself—in order to find the strength and will to take care of him. Sometimes that may mean saying no to him or others when they stress you needlessly, and yes to things you need for yourself.

PLAYING THE HAND YOU'RE DEALT

YES, OF COURSE women get sick, too, as they age, but women tend to get sick later in life than men. Although the life-expectancy gender gap has narrowed a bit, on average we still live more than five years longer than our men. In addition, women often marry or have relationships with men who are older than they are. There's no getting around it: far more often we must take care of our men than vice versa. Most of us are still probably hardwired to be caregivers. In all my years of practice I can't remember a woman, no matter how successful, who didn't know somewhere in her brain where her husband or children were at a given time. Few men have a similar mind-set.

Despite these truths, taking care of an ailing spouse is a role change you never wanted or asked for. It's a shift that affects every aspect of your life, including your marriage or committed relationship, your emotional and financial security, and the very foundation of your family. And when you become a caregiver to your partner, the goal is to do more than just survive. It's to live as full a life as possible, even when the quality of his life is compromised. It's to function effectively, using your strengths to achieve what you must and accept that you aren't perfect and will never be. I will show you how.

HOW TO USE THIS BOOK

MY INTENTION is that you can pick up this book at any time and turn to an appropriate chapter for insight, practical information, comfort, reassurance, or support. You do not have to read *When the Man You Love Is Ill* from beginning to end in one sitting. However, if there is time, I do recommend reading chapters 2 and 3 first, to help you focus and feel less inadequate and alone.

Here's how to find what you need quickly:

- In an emergency or crisis:

  You have lots of information needs. Chapter 7 helps you become an instant expert on your mate's condition. Then you can make the most informed decisions possible when you're in a tough spot. Chapter 8 helps you become an advocate for him and a liaison between him and the doctors and the medical system. At the same time, your fear and panic can interfere with effective action. Chapter 13 helps you cope with these and other feelings. If you're also holding the family together, see chapter 5. Chapter 9 can be useful for job-related issues, such as notifying your partner's boss and checking out health insurance coverage.

- During extended treatment, recuperation, or post-treatment:

  Read chapter 2 to become aware of what it takes to be an effective support for your man, as well as a loving one. In chapter 3 you can identify your personal coping style in times of adversity and pinpoint your strengths and areas that need work. He may have adjustment issues, decisions about going back to work, or depression. Chapter 6 helps you help him by understanding why men behave the way they do when they are sick.

New insights can help you become more patient with him and head off anger or irritation. Conflict between the two of you has a negative effect on his healing. See chapters 10, 11, and 12 to protect your couple relationship and deal with sexual issues. Chapter 4 helps you gather support from family and other sources, including support groups.

- In a long-term chronic illness:

    If you're troubled by what you consider shameful or disturbing thoughts creeping into your head, in chapter 13 you'll discover that you are not alone. That same chapter can help you deal with anxiety, guilt, and other emotions. Chapters 4 and 13 help you prevent burnout during years of caregiving, and chapter 14 offers ways to protect your own health. Turn to chapters 10, 11, and 12 to help you deal with inevitable stresses and painful issues in your relationship, to stay close, and if possible, to move toward transformational love.

    See chapter 4 for information on face-to-face and online caregiver support groups. Chapter 7 helps you keep up with the latest treatment advances and educate yourself to changes in your mate's condition.

- When it's terminal:

    Facing a partner's death is a complex and devastating experience. Chapter 15 helps you through the important decisions—and life ahead.

Note that chapter 16 offers advice for men who are taking care of ill spouses. You may wish to show it to a male friend who is struggling with caregiving issues.

Each chapter has much to offer, and I hope you will finish the entire book at some point. But you don't have to read in any particular order. Just go ahead and gather bits of what you need as you need them.

Reflections

- *Sometimes life knocks you down, but it is possible to pick yourself up and get through it.*

- *There is nothing noble about sacrificing your health and well-being.*

- *Virtually everyone in your shoes feels scared and overwhelmed.*

- *You don't have to do everything yourself.*

- *In tough times, you can strengthen your relationship.*

2

Becoming an
Effective Support

Dear Annie,

I am sitting here in the office, but all I can think about is how wonderful you are. I truly do not deserve someone like you. You make me want to feel better and are more disappointed than I am if I don't.

This morning when you started to cry because you didn't search the Internet earlier, it broke my heart. I know how much you want life to return to normal and that we are in this together.

I love you more than words can say. Things will get better.

A grateful husband wrote these words to his wife after she found a product online that dramatically improved the quality of his life. For months she had watched helplessly as an agonizing skin irritation wore him down. It developed after cancer treatment, and nothing suggested by the doctor relieved the pain. Her husband had tried everything—from over-the-counter ointments to a special formulation at forty-two dollars per tube—but to no avail.

In desperation, Annie finally turned to the Internet and undertook her own research, hoping to find a remedy. She discovered a cream that seemed ideal and checked with the doctor to make sure the ingredients were safe for her husband's situation. The cream not only soothed the pain, it banished the problem completely after several weeks of use.

The point of the story is this: It takes love plus effective behavior to help your mate when he is suffering. Annie's love compelled her to persist in her search. Taking care of your partner effectively and thoughtfully means giving him (or getting him) the help he needs—in whatever form it takes. It also means using good judgment, not just acting impulsively because you're scared. In some situations, quick thinking or assertiveness makes the difference; in others, as in Annie's case, it's patience, flexibility, or persistence. The exact nature of effective behavior depends on what's going on, which can change as time passes. When a condition worsens, for example, causing your mate to become less self-sufficient, your own physical stamina becomes an issue. If there is a perfect woman somewhere who is good at meeting all of the demands that can arise, I've never met her.

Many of my clients have managed to do what they must—and more. In the process they have reached a place of self-acceptance. Over time, they have come to understand they are "good enough" at providing necessary care. It is possible for you, too, to be good enough, by understanding what it takes and learning to handle your own unsettling feelings. Strategies that have worked for my clients can also help you.

YOUR EMOTIONAL LANDSCAPE

ANNIE EXPERIENCED A number of uncomfortable emotions as she struggled with her mate's care, and you may, too. When providing care, virtually all of us experience feelings such as these at times:

- Fear
- Anger
- Anxiety
- Ambivalence
- Helplessness
- Confusion

These powerful feelings may be unwanted, and they may show themselves in ways that are new to you. When ignored or denied, they may hinder you in doing all that you have to do. If your partner's illness forces major changes in your life or lifestyle, other feelings may take effect over the longer period, such as depression, resentment, frustration, sadness, loneliness, and guilt. These, too, are normal and not a cause for shame. They are certainly not a reason to withdraw from those people who are available to help you.

As I work with caregivers in crisis, I try to help them deal with *all* of their emotions, no matter how unwelcome they are. By acknowledging and confronting negative feelings, it can become easier to function in spite of them. You may not be able to change your mate's medical condition, but you do have control over your response to it.

SEVEN ELEMENTS OF EFFECTIVE CARE

I'VE FOUND THAT effective behavior when your mate is ill (and you are scared, sad, mad, or overwhelmed) involves components that are rarely examined. I call these components "the seven C's." They can help you to understand more about what constitutes effective action in your situation—and provide goals to strive for.

Try to keep the seven C's on your radar screen as you go about the business of supporting your mate. They are:

1. **Communication.** It's crucial to talk honestly with medical personnel, family, and friends—and the most important person, your partner. Much as we would like, few people are mind readers. Yet it's common to expect other people to know our thoughts without any input from us. We may think, "He (or she) should know. I shouldn't have to spell it out." But communicating exactly what's on your mind is important.

   I often tell clients, "My degree is in psychology; I'm not a psychic. You need to tell me what you're thinking and feeling." The clearer you articulate questions and concerns, the easier it will be to get the right help from doctors, nurses, relatives, and friends. Remember, too, that talking things out with your mate (if his condition permits) can lead to creative problem solving and can draw you closer together. You can become a better team.

2. **Compassion.** Research shows that support from a spouse is the most important kind when your partner is sick. When you are aware of his pain and suffering and able to empathize, you bring him solace and strength. Be aware, however, that empathy is *not* the same as getting totally absorbed in his experience—which helps nobody. Naturally, you want to know why he walks around moaning, and you imagine what he is going through. But the goal is to understand his pain rather than be compelled to feel it yourself. Living in his skin only drains and debilitates you. You run the risk of losing yourself when he needs you to be a separate person, someone who can think and act objectively on his behalf.

3. **Connection.** Conversation and touch help keep us alive. I recall a client who woke up after major surgery. The first words he spoke to his wife were, "Give me a hug." Since tubes were in the way, she did the next best thing and caressed his face. The gesture told him eloquently, "I'm still here and I love you."

   A hand on his shoulder or the back of his neck, or a pat on the back, reassures him he's loved and gives him a sense of security at a time when he feels helpless and vulnerable. It's powerful medicine.

   Try to pay attention to your own need for connection and support, and maintain contact with your social network. Isolation is a danger to your health and well-being and weakens your resilience.

4. **Conflict.** There's no escaping internal conflict and ambivalence about the burden your partner's condition may impose on you and the way it has changed your life. In an intense long-term situation, as time goes on you may feel so overwhelmed by his needs that it's hard to remember why you love him (or that you ever did).

   "Disaster is always on my doorstep," says Delores. "I seem to spend my life listening to sounds from the bedroom that mean he's in trouble." It can be very painful to voice such seemingly negative yet normal thoughts, but try it. Acknowledgment dilutes the guilt you may feel for thinking such things.

   It's reassuring to realize that many other people have struggled with the same feelings. This path is yours alone, but it has been walked by others before.

5. **Courage.** It's hard to stand up to uncertainty, not knowing whether he'll have a recurrence, when the next attack will occur, or how long he'll be able to work. It's also difficult

to learn more about his medical condition and what it portends in your life—and to learn about yourself. It takes a brave soul to venture into the unknown and face whatever may come. True, a certain amount of denial can be healthy at times and get you through. Denial becomes destructive if it stops you from taking important next steps, such as investigating treatment options.

When you feel fear, you also have the opportunity to experience courage. Think of it this way: there is always a tension between the psychological "comfort zone"—the desire to remain in control—and the dense fog of the unknown ahead. Try to anticipate and accept fear as normal and natural in this tough situation. That acceptance can bring tremendous relief and help you to prevail.

6. **Cooperation.** To get through your caregiving experience, find ways to work productively with medical staff, your partner (if possible), and everyone else in your life. Keep your eye on the goal, whether it's getting him to the emergency room, facilitating his recovery, easing his pain, or figuring out how to get test results tomorrow instead of next week. For the moment, try to put aside emotions, such as anger, that may interfere with accomplishing that goal.

For example, you may want to blow up at the doctor's rude receptionist, but that probably won't get you what you want. You have a much better chance for a productive result if you swallow your impulse to swat her and instead ask, "What can I do to help you speed things along?"

Hard as it may be, the same advice applies to interactions with family members. You need their help. This is a time to put aside any differences you have in order to work together for the greater good—the health and well-being of your mate. For example, a client I'll call Wendy had a domineering older sister whose condescending tone made her wince. Wendy realized that her sister's bossiness could be an asset in gathering information from medical staff, and she put her to work. On balance, the benefits of her sister's help outweighed the irritations. In addition, her sister felt needed and valued.

When possible, teamwork between you and your partner—the idea that "We're in this together"—is enormously useful. This attitude brings you closer, and two heads working together *are* better than one. However, if his fear or anger about his situation boils over, he may not have it in him to cooperate. He may even fight you, making your already tough job even tougher. At such times it helps to understand why he behaves that way. Chapter 6 offers insights and positive suggestions for dealing with his issues.

7. **Control.** In this case, the definition of control is to manage what you can, organize, and take charge of what you can realistically do. Control does not imply being stoic or doing everything yourself. It does mean that when it comes to decisions your partner can't make for himself, the buck usually stops with you.

The seven C's add up to a formidable "awareness" list. The idea is to use them piece by piece. You can't absorb all the C's (let alone act upon them) immediately. Give yourself time, and realize that in a particular situation some C's may be more essential than others. Focusing on the C's will help you stay centered, pay attention to your feelings and strengths, and think about effective action.

IT'S OKAY TO BE YOURSELF

THE PROCESS OF becoming "good enough" is never a straight line. You have to gradually become comfortable with the seven C's and at the same time fight off self-criticism and fear of failure when you're beleaguered by caregiving demands. It may be hard to resist taking action merely to stave off anxiety. For example, you may not want to take the time for a second opinion. Yet it is possible to slow down, weigh the pros and cons, and make careful, reasoned decisions.

It is also possible to handle your mate and his illness in your own personal way—and be who you are, as you are. Although you may feel under duress and defeated at times, your way can be very effective. If you need help, run, do not walk, to your most trusted source of support.

Reflections

- *"Good enough" is indeed good enough to help him.*

- *Acknowledge unwelcome emotions such as anger, fear, and guilt. You can learn to handle them.*

- *Be alert to the seven C's: communication, compassion, connection, conflict, courage, cooperation, and control.*

- *Take the time to focus on one or two of the seven C's to improve your situation.*

- *Remember, you can't be anybody else. Your way is okay.*

3

What's Your Coping Style?

"*I discovered that* you can do anything, including dressing wounds that only nurses used to tend," says Bonnie, who took care of her husband after several of his hospitalizations. "Sure, you get terrified and think you'll faint, but you do what you have to, because among other things, your insurance will cover only so many home care visits. The home nurse trains you, although it's never long enough for your peace of mind. At first you can barely stand to look at the incision. But after the first few times, you do become accustomed to it. You even get good at it and start feeling proud of yourself. You're stronger than you think."

It's frightening when your mate's well-being, or even his very life, depends on what you do. The responsibility is suddenly so great. If you think at first that you'll never get it right, try not to fret. Whether you're giving him injections or acting as an advocate to get him the best care, it takes time to feel your way.

Now that you know the components of effective caregiving—the seven C's—the goal is to give your abilities room to grow. We all possess undeveloped potential. Although your first thought might be, "I could never do *that*," impossible as it may seem right now, you may ultimately discover otherwise. A good way to become more capable is to understand how you function and react to events in your life. I've found in my years of practice that clients cope with adversity in significantly different ways. The following assessment will help you identify your own coping style and understand how you deal with your mate's condition.

WHAT'S YOUR COPING STYLE?

LIKE ALL OF us, you have your own way of being in the world. Your personality traits affect how you perceive relationships and situations. Your attitudes influence and help shape your experience. As a result, the way you handle adversity will affect your caregiving.

To identify your coping style, circle the answers below that seem to fit you best. Keep in mind that no one style is the best style or your only style. Each has advantages and disadvantages.

1. The group of adjectives that best describes me is:
   a. Practical, realistic, analytical, proactive
   b. Compassionate, intuitive, sensitive, emotional
   c. Idealistic, spiritual, faithful, philosophical

2. When I make an important decision, I usually:
   a. Think through the pluses and minuses of each choice and how each will affect me
   b. Consider the position of everyone involved and choose the option that creates the most harmony
   c. Meditate and let the answers come to me

3. When I am in a crisis, I:
   a. Believe in acting first and pushing my emotions into the background
   b. Feel and then do
   c. Remind myself that everything happens for a reason

4. If there is a conflict at work or home, I:
   a. Take action and find solutions—and let the chips fall where they may
   b. Am empathetic first and try to sense what others may want
   c. Believe things will work out for the best

5. When I am in a bad mood, I:
   a. Do something productive, such as clean my desk or go to the gym
   b. Give myself a break and call a friend or family member to talk
   c. Take a walk and wait for the answer to become clear

6. When I am ill, I want:
   a. To take action to get better
   b. To be catered to or left alone with my feelings
   c. To seek inner peace however I can, such as through meditation and prayer

7. If I see an automobile accident, I am most likely to:
   a. Whip out my cell phone and call 911 (or ask someone else to do it)
   b. Feel so anxious that my head swims and my gut knots; I'm paralyzed
   c. Stay calm and pray for the victims' health

8. When dealing with someone in authority who has power over me and dislikes me, I:
   a. Talk to him/her about how we can work more productively together, or say, "Can you tell me what the problem is? I'd like to solve it."
   b. Feel hurt or angry enough to want to hit back or seek revenge
   c. Pray for the person or turn the other cheek

9. The saying that appeals most to me is:
   a. "When the going gets rough, it's time to get tough."
   b. "Love conquers all."
   c. "I am part of a greater plan."

10. When confronted with a family dilemma, I:
    a. Write out a list of things I can do to help
    b. Consider my feelings and ask other family members how they feel about it
    c. Believe in destiny and miracles

INTERPRETING YOUR RESULTS

I'VE FOUND THAT clients tend to use one of three dominant coping styles. They are what I call "thinkers," "feelers," or "believers." If you circled mostly A's, you tend to be a "thinker." Mostly B's, you're usually a "feeler." Mostly C's, you're generally a "believer."

The explanations that follow will help you understand your own primary coping style. Once you know how you operate in the world, you can begin to pinpoint your strengths and identify behaviors you can modify to make life better for you and your mate. You may also deal more effectively with anxiety and other emotions that can interfere with caregiving.

If You're a Thinker:

If you're a thinker, you're someone who tends to be logical and goal-oriented and who reasons things through. (For example, managers are often thinkers.) You target the problem at hand and immediately ask, "What can we do now?" When your mate is seriously ill, you tend to focus on finding solutions.

Upside: You usually function well in crises and emergencies when quick decisions must be made. Fear and other immobilizing emotions are pushed out of your consciousness and put on the back burner when your mate is in jeopardy. You get results and are probably a good information gatherer. You want to know everything you can about an illness and how to cure or treat it. Because you're pragmatic, you also may be good at performing demanding medical tasks.

Downside: When things aren't going well, you may become impatient and lose sight of your mate's emotions and preferences when decisions must be made. You also may resist help when offered, believing you are ultimately responsible for his care. Afraid of giving up control, you can wear yourself out trying to do it all. Your blood pressure may soar off the charts.

Areas to work on: When you are stressed, empathy and compassion may not be your strong suits. Most people start out feeling compassion when disaster strikes, but some don't know how to express it, or they get so worn down they may snap at their partner. If you don't feel very compassionate toward your mate, it's frequently because you tend to intellectualize what is happening. You probably set strict priorities. He spills his drink; you clean up the mess without a thought to how *he* may feel—inadequate, embarrassed, ashamed, and needing reassurance from you. When he forgets a step in trying to dress his own wound, you may demand, "Can't you get it right?" Unfortunately, you're so busy getting things done that empathy gets lost.

You don't feel good about yourself in such situations, and although it's only human to be short-tempered at times, it isn't good for either of you. To keep such lapses to a minimum, notice when you're feeling harassed and unsympathetic. Constant problem solving may stress you out and lead you to act insensitively. When you're wound up tight, you can have a more difficult time connecting emotionally with your mate.

As a thinker, you may need to slow down and try to fight against your tendency to ignore intuition and body warning signals. Take exhaustion, headaches, backaches, and other symptoms of stress seriously. So many proud and/or successful people develop resistance to help and wind up getting depressed. Try to break through such patterns. You may not be able to do this alone.

If You're a Feeler:

If you're a feeler, you are "gut smart." You pay attention to your own (and other people's) feelings. You tend to your mate with compassion and affection. You know intuitively that "he needs a hug." You may realize that a particular doctor is the wrong person to treat your mate without being able to articulate exactly why.

Feelers are complicated, however. Although many can be wonderfully compassionate and giving souls, others become so overwhelmed by feelings that they function erratically or not at all. Generally, feelers fit one of these descriptions or the other.

Upside: You probably make a good caregiver if you're a feeler with a natural tendency to nurture, comfort, and console. You're empathetic and automatically try to put yourself in others' shoes. As a result, you may excel at day-to-day caregiving and tolerate well the demands of a long-term illness. Some feelers rise to heights of generosity and instinctively know when a mate needs a sip of water or even when a hospital nurse needs a cup of coffee. In addition, you often involve other people in your mate's illness and may be more willing to let others help. You know how to get the best out of medical personnel.

Downside: If you're a compassionate feeler, you may be lax about exploring options for your mate. You may hesitate to ask whether the ambulance can take him to the best emergency room rather than simply the nearest one. You may also prefer to avoid confrontation or conflict. You may lack the courage to stand up to a misguided medical professional. It may be difficult to say no to your mate when he tries to manipulate you or when he overestimates his own physical stamina.

If you're a feeler whose emotions overwhelm you in a crisis, you aren't able to act as effectively as is needed. "I get such anxiety that it affects my cognitive ability. I can't think. I actually become stupid," explains Emily, whose partner has coped with kidney cancer and arthritis. On the other hand, some overwhelmed feelers can become so emotional they may lash out at the nearest target.

Areas to work on: You may have to call on others to stand by you in acute situations where you're apt to be overwhelmed and need help with problem-solving skills or goal setting. If you're just too scattered to reason properly, find someone else who can tend to details and pitch in with other aid. Sometimes feelers need a therapist or confidant to help sort out priorities and feelings and to advise, "You have to think things through."

Compassionate feelers can experience the patient's stress as if it were their own. If you're one of them, you run the risk of making yourself sick. You may need professional help to cope with out-of-control emotions, such as frequent crying in your mate's presence.

If You're a Believer:

If you tend to be a believer, you may or may not worship God or belong to an organized religion. But you do believe in fate and destiny, and you have faith that the answers will come to you. You may be well equipped to lend calm and strength to your mate at a time when he desperately needs both. For example, you may view his heart attack as "meant to be" rather than a catastrophe. You may be able to take your time to make thoughtful decisions.

Upside: When confronted with adversity, your fundamental faith that everything happens for a reason may help you roll with the punches. You're likely to remain calm rather than panic, and you probably respond to bad news with "How can I rise to the occasion?" or "How do I grow into this new role?" or "What is the meaning behind this event?" Because you may believe what happens is for the best, you can offer equanimity and peace that is experienced as healing by your mate.

You may also have a built-in community at your disposal, with help readily available through your place of worship. You probably use the support system of clergy and fellow parishioners willingly and well. You may also be open to alternative medical treatments. Statements like "Pray for him" or "Send healing energy his way" may come easily to you.

Downside: In a medical crisis, your deep faith may lead you to play a passive role because you believe what is meant to be will happen on its own. You may throw up your hands, say, "It's God's will," and forget that you still have to make decisions.

Medically important details that could help or hurt your mate may be ignored. You may believe the universe helps those who help themselves. As a result, you may want to do everything yourself and reject useful help.

Catastrophe can sometimes shake faith temporarily or even permanently. People may go through a personal crisis of their own. If this happens to you, your personal support systems can be in jeopardy.

Areas to work on: You're likely to have trouble with conflict and may withdraw rather than deal with it. Make an effort to seek information—don't hesitate to get a second opinion or find information on drug trials if it could benefit your mate. Draw on your "thinker" side and set priorities. (Conversely, a thinker may need to turn off the power switch and get more in touch with her spiritual side. Without quiet time to refuel, it's easy to burn out.)

REMEMBER, NONE OF the three coping styles is the perfect one. People are complex and have more than one way of coping. Yet you probably lean toward one dominant style. Sometimes you may flow from one style to another as your mate's illness pushes you to use every talent you have. And you may surprise yourself with how well you do. I've seen some people rise to new heights and pull hitherto unknown rabbits out of hats.

For example, Maxine, an insecure driver who always preferred others to take the wheel, performed a feat of heroism to help her husband, a cancer survivor. While the couple was on vacation in Vermont, he developed an excruciatingly painful infection. Maxine was able to reach his doctor, who called in an antibiotic prescription to the closest pharmacy. The pharmacy was twenty miles away over narrow mountain roads, and it was already dark. "I was shaking all the way, but somehow I forced myself to make the round trip to get the medication. My husband was in agony and I had no choice. I'm still amazed I was able to do it," says Maxine.

However, at least initially, it's natural to lean on those behaviors that are most comfortable and familiar to you. If you naturally solve problems, that's what you will tend to do when he's sick. You're a thinker. It makes sense. We are creatures of habit. At times of stress, however, it's common to get stuck in habits that may not be useful. For example, you may be accustomed to barking orders to get things done. But your softer side may serve you (and your mate) better during a setback in a long recuperation, where all you can do is wait and hope that lost ground will be recovered.

I hope you will view your coping style as an asset and as a road map that, once understood, helps you lean on your strengths, recognize situations where you function best, and come to terms with the challenges you face. These insights will help you move farther along the path to self-acceptance and taking care of your partner effectively.

SIX WAYS TO EXPAND YOUR COPING STYLE

ALTHOUGH YOU MAY be predominantly a thinker, a feeler, or a believer, you possess many dimensions. To uncover the wider range of your own potential and function more fully:

1. **Remember, no one is perfect.**

    Don't expect to excel at everything. I don't know of anyone who is both a relentless advocate for her mate *and* a model of patience and nurturing *and* an oasis of spiritual peace. Do you? Try not to become a harsh, unforgiving judge. Be kind to yourself, or you'll never get through this. The goal is to use your strengths and get help for your challenges, which each and every one of us has.

2. Notice the situations that are most difficult for you.

Try to stay aware of them. For example, my client Patty automatically panics when her mate is ill or injured. Her emotions take center stage, and she spills and vents. She feels so squeamish and intimidated by medical technology that she has a meltdown if asked to apply ointment and a gauze pad. Instead of dealing with her fear at such times, she may get angry. Some people must take care not to use anger or denial as a smoke-screen for feeling inadequate or afraid.

Don't expect to feel confident right away. It takes practice to achieve the feeling of "good enough" competence. You do have to fight off self-criticism and fear of failure. What seems awkward and impossible at first often becomes doable eventually.

3. Ask others to check out your coping skills.

If self-assessment isn't one of your strengths, or you feel too overwhelmed to be objective, you may need help in judging your coping capabilities (or lack thereof). Sometimes your perception of yourself may differ from the view of those you most trust and love. It may help to see if their assessment of you coincides with your own—and if you're up to it, discuss any differences.

Talk with a close friend, a sibling, or a cousin—any person who knows you very well and has your best interests at heart. Someone else may be able to say, "You're not good at details" or "You tend to lose your head in a crisis" or "You seem depressed. You may need medication."

When you see yourself as others see you, it's easier to think about your caregiving personality and make changes in behavior. For example, if you're proactive and competent, you may need to consider hiring an aide in a long-term situation or ask family members to pitch in because you're also impatient.

4. Do what you have to do to function.

Some women, usually the feelers and believers, find solace in spending twelve hours a day (or twenty-four) at the hospital feeling useful and watchful. Florence was not among them when her husband had a stroke years ago. Her limit was three hours a day (plus a forty-five-minute commute each way). "That was all I could take. The more time I spent in a dreary waiting room or at a bedside, the closer I drifted toward depression. I timed my arrival for just after the doctors had completed morning rounds, when they could report on my husband's condition. He wasn't paralyzed, but he had lost expressive function. He not only couldn't speak, he couldn't read, or write his own name," she says.

Florence spent the rest of the day reassuring two sets of elderly parents (his and hers), being there for her two teenage sons, returning phone calls, and checking the hospital for updates. Fortunately, her husband made a full recovery and was able to return to his law practice four months later. Her tolerance has increased since then. She's an example of a woman who has grown.

"I'm more experienced now and therefore less likely to panic. I've learned a lot and matured. The first or second time major illness happens, you feel terrified, whether or not you show it. Inside, you may think you're going to collapse. By the third or fourth time, you know you can get through it somehow—because you already have," she explains.

With experience also came the ability to live in the moment instead of obsessing about problems down the road. "'Take one day at a time,' which sometimes seems like a bromide, really is good advice. Focusing on the here and now helps you cope in bite-sized pieces and feel less overwhelmed," she says.

Another wife managed to stay sane in her own inimitable way. She went shopping while her husband was in surgery. Like Dorothy in *The Wizard of Oz,* she was transported by the magic of her new shoes. Others go to the gym, see a movie, get a massage, or take the kids to McDonald's to escape. The point is that most short-term distractions are positive if they're legal, don't hurt anyone, and keep you from falling apart.

Of course, for many people, especially believers, prayer can be an enormous help and comfort. So is asking others to pray for your partner. You can never have too many people rooting for you.

5. Give yourself time to learn.

Stretching your capabilities doesn't happen instantly. You didn't go to nursing school, and it takes time and practice to build expertise. You may wish to consider getting caregiver training. There's a right way and a wrong way to lift a person, for example, and improving other skills can save wear and tear on you and the patient. If your mate has diabetes, appropriate training in self-care and overcoming problems educates him and you. Medicare (and some private insurance) covers it.

For example, the Joslin Diabetes Center, based in Boston, offers workshops for couples or individual diabetics at its many U.S. locations. Some general caregiver training is available through local chapters of the Red Cross. The Center for Caregiver Training offers free online training (www.caregiving101.org). You can also type the words "caregiver training" into an Internet search engine, such as Google, for other resources.

Although caregiving training programs are usually geared to caring for elderly parents, much information can also apply to a mate.

6. **Realize that the past influences the present.**

Not many people take caregiving courses. Most learned their modes of caregiving while growing up and watching family members tend to the ill. Patterns that you saw at home influence your own behavior as an adult. You may embrace these patterns or rebel against them. If you saw nurturing, compassionate caregiving, you already have a blueprint for that kind of behavior and are more likely to do the same. If not, you have to invent your own blueprint.

Perhaps your mother gave up her career to care for your ill father and wound up becoming a bitter woman and a destructive, intrusive caregiver. You may be determined not to follow these footsteps. And if you stay aware, you have a better chance of changing that pattern. Maybe your father lovingly cared for your mother during years of on-and-off illness. You remember that he also took time-outs for himself. He told you, "I love your mother, but life goes on." That attitude may sustain you now. Or perhaps your aunt made herself a doormat while caring for your sick uncle. You don't want that to happen to you.

ACCEPT REALITY

THRUST INTO A situation where you have no choice, you're probably far more capable than you realize in areas where you've always felt inadequate. Emily, the anxious "feeler," calls herself "a recovering panicker." She has learned to ask for help when she's too overwhelmed to act by herself; she has also learned to calm and soothe herself so that she can think. She takes care of business. "You gotta find a way," she says.

The fact is, nobody's good at everything, and it takes time to extend your reach. With practice and determination, many of my clients have not only learned new skills, they've felt a sense of mastery, which leads to greater emotional stability.

It is also true, however, that some people never develop their caregiving skills. If you're one of them, accept that about yourself. Going to work may be an emotional refuge for you. It may make sense to pay someone else to take care of your mate if you can afford it. If money is tight, see page 147 for information on options. Use your unique strengths to do what you must to get through this difficult challenge.

Reflections

- *Take pride in what you can do.*

- *Understand that practice and experience help you become more capable in areas where you're needed.*

- *Identify your primary coping style. Use your strengths and get help for your challenges.*

- *Realize that there is no single ideal coping style and that you are capable of using more than one. Each has advantages and disadvantages.*

- *Remember, nobody's good at everything.*

4

Reaching Out for Help

"I have three neighbors who also have sick husbands and know just what I'm going through. We meet every day at the mailboxes to trade stories and tips on everything from dealing with doctors (and our husbands' moods) to patient-friendly gadgets that make life easier. We don't socialize anywhere else, but we help each other a lot. It's always better to talk to someone who understands," says Noreen, from Portland, Oregon.

When your partner, the closest person in your life, is ill, you desperately need community and the support of other people. My personal mantra, and the theme of my Web site, www.Fiftyand Furthermore.com, is "Life is too hard to do alone. Reach out." I use this mantra as a reminder that connection with others is a lifeline for all of us. This is true especially in an age when distance separates many families and friends, and when those who are close by live increasingly busy lives.

Research confirms the assertion of the seventeenth-century poet John Donne: "No man is an island." We are less healthy than we could be and live a shortened life span when we lack a loving, intimate relationship and a close community. We can't fully thrive without meaningful contact with others. When you're feeling under siege, one answer is to reach out.

Proceed with caution, of course. Not everyone is worthy of trust. The idea is to open up to people you can rely on and those professionals you value. Welcome aid from unexpected sources instead of automatically dismissing it. Sometimes the best help shows up in surprising packages.

REACHING OUT MAY BE DIFFICULT

UNLESS YOU'VE SPENT your life hidden away from society (or meditating on a mountain), chances are you never realized that you've always lived in a group. You and your mate and, by extension, your family are the most important group in your life. Hopefully you are also part of other groups, such as your neighborhood, town or city, religious affiliation, the children's schools, or work.

Your partner's illness has dealt a major blow to your special life-sustaining group—the two of you within your marriage or significant relationship. To withstand the assault and still function as you must, you need help. Other groups in your life can often provide it, but you may have to overcome resistance to asking for aid.

Like many people, you may have been brought up to believe that telling anyone about personal matters is wrong. You may have heard messages such as "Don't air your dirty laundry in public." "No one is interested in what you do." "What goes on in the family stays in the family." If that was the family philosophy, reaching out for support not only goes against your grain, it's something you don't know how to do. Or maybe your early life experiences taught you that when you ask for help, you'll be rejected. Others will say no. You've learned they won't come through for you, so asking just seems too painful to risk.

Whether or not you are accustomed to seeking support, this is a time to do so. A mate's serious illness shakes up everything that has been stable and sustaining in your life. Few of us can manage the rigors alone.

QUIZ: HOW DO I FEEL ABOUT REACHING OUT?

Answer True or False to the statements below to help gauge your own attitude about asking for and accepting help:

1. People who ask for assistance are weak.

_____ True   _____ False

2. Asking for help obligates you to others, and I don't want to be beholden to anyone.

_____ True   _____ False

3. I'd rather not ask for help than take the risk of being rejected.

_____ True   _____ False

4 People should take care of their own without help.

_____ True   _____ False

5. Family matters should always remain private.

_____ True   _____ False

If you answered True for three or more of these statements, you may be trying to do too much alone and even be heading for trouble. Your task is to stay healthy and be the most generous and effective caregiver you can be. Ask yourself, "Can I really do this alone? Or will my mate and family do better with extra support?"

FAMILY RESOURCES

NEWS OF A serious diagnosis can have a powerful effect on your extended family. Hopefully, it draws kin together. When this happens, the family may be a welcoming shelter, offering warmth and willing practical support. However, family can also feel like a chaotic intrusion. Relatives may bombard you with questions about your partner's condition and what they can do to help, which amounts to asking you to manage *them* at a time when you're already reeling from all you have to do.

A family meeting is one way to organize and involve extended family members and get much-needed assistance. It takes some of the pressure off you when you can get input from a variety of people and discuss what needs to be done. Of course, you want to include only family members you trust, respect, and feel comfortable with. If bringing these people together has the potential to cause a family rift—as when Uncle Joe is important to you, but you can't stand his wife—you may have to reach for an extra dose of tolerance. Don't forget your mate's siblings and parents or, if yours is a blended family, your stepson or stepdaughter.

Under the stress of an emergency, it may be too difficult for you to coordinate everyone. In that case, you can appoint someone as a surrogate manager to direct all the "troops." Delegating doesn't mean you don't love your mate or have lost control. It does mean you use available resources and conserve precious energy for those tasks that only you can do. Delegating also delivers another benefit: the appointee feels useful, and his or her participation can actually knit the family together.

Whether the manager is you or someone else, the idea is to assign the best roles and match people to appropriate tasks. Perhaps your cousin Clyde is a gifted gardener who can keep the yard looking neat and attractive. Someone else may be able to take your mate to the dentist or stay with him while you attend the PTA meeting. When you ask people to do what they do best, you can transform their potentially annoying personality traits into assets. Maybe your cousin Betty is smart and computer savvy but has a grating habit of endlessly asking questions. She may be the perfect choice to research medical information. Perhaps your sibling can visit your elderly mother more often, freeing you to spend more time on your husband's or children's needs. A little creativity can go a long way.

I remember one couple who had to cope with the husband's liver cancer diagnosis. They were blessed with a psychologically astute sister-in-law, who left her three children with her husband in Chicago so that she could fly to Massachusetts to help. This woman organized and led the family meeting, asking people what they could do best.

A niece ferried the patient's elderly parents back and forth to the hospital from their hotel. A cousin prepared food and brought games and books to keep the anxious relatives occupied. Her sense of humor became a much-needed tonic that relieved tension in the family lounge during the wait for news of the cancer surgery. At one point she even put on a clown face, triggering a round of giggles and guffaws.

I think of this family as a role model of supportive effort. They didn't always get along, but when catastrophe struck, past hurts were set aside. Support came first.

There are so many ways people can be useful. For example, it's exhausting to give updates to everyone. You can feel like a broken record. In one family the wife's sister took over the chore. She happened to be a congenial person and a good writer. She fielded the deluge of e-mails, cards, and telephone calls from friends and coworkers—and filtered those that her brother-in-law and sister would want to read for themselves. Periodically, she sent updates to an organized list. At the end of the day, she sat with the patient, listening to his distress when necessary, and helping him unwind and even talk sports.

Sometimes family members take their help a step further. In one case, a brother donated a kidney for a transplant. A sister closed her business a thousand miles away and arrived to help. "My own brother came for two weeks with his girlfriend, who was wonderful. What a gift!" says the wife.

Unfortunately, not everyone has relatives to turn to. Some families are unsupportive or even downright destructive. Certain clients have told me, "My family is the last place I'd go for help." If that's your situation, there may be other sources of assistance outside the family that you haven't considered.

FRIENDS AND COMMUNITY

OFTEN, PRACTICAL HELP, as well as solace, is available from churches, synagogues, and other places of worship. Part of their mission is providing aid to the ill and their families. Many congregations have committees or specific volunteers who deal with the sick or those in financial need.

Members of two local churches in Missouri helped sustain Lorraine, a mother of two preschoolers, when her husband faced a bone marrow transplant. Hearing of her plight, parishioners offered this: "Put a cooler on your front porch, and we'll deliver meals every day. We'll call to tell you what we're making."

Lorraine recalls, "They filled that cooler every day for nine months, and they weren't even my denomination." She admits that she never would have considered this kind of aid before, but she accepted it gratefully. "We women have a hard time asking for help. We're like men who so often refuse to ask for directions. We think we have to do it all, but we can't."

More help arrived when her husband was ready to come home from the hospital. "Because he had no immune system, the entire house had to be disinfected in advance, following a thirty-six-page manual of cleaning instructions. Two church volunteers, my parents, a friend, and I worked at it for over one hundred hours. At first it was overwhelming, but it became doable with our 'clean team,'" she says.

Local generosity also amazed another wife, whose husband battled advanced kidney disease. Neighbors took up a collection for this mother of three, presenting her with gift certificates for the local supermarket.

At the same time that strangers can be enormously helpful, some family relationships and friendships may change when your mate is seriously ill, especially if the illness goes on for a long time. Creeping isolation is all too common as a disease progresses or treatment continues for months or years. People stop coming around, because they don't know what to say or do, or because taking care of your mate takes up more and more of your time. They can drift away if you can't participate in social activities the way you used to. I always urge clients to recognize who the most helpful people are and to realize that they may be different from those they were close to before. For example, a tennis partner with the knack for offering specific help becomes solid gold when she says, "I can come right over to sit with you at the hospital. Would you like that?"

Other Random Acts of Kindness

Support may also turn up in unusual places if you speak up and tell others what's going on. For example, one of my clients, Randi, whose husband had severe emphysema, regularly attended a yoga class. One day she mentioned the stress in her life to the other women in the locker room. Everyone immediately responded, "How can we help?"—and they proceeded to form a network to assist her. At first she felt shy about asking for something specific and was a little bit overwhelmed.

Finally, unable to think, she replied, "What do you have in mind?"

A great deal, as it happened. Randi's yoga group decided it would be easier for her if they came to her home for yoga instruction so that she wouldn't have to travel. One person, a professional massage therapist, offered to give her a relaxing massage every week. The rest volunteered to stay with her children as needed. Suddenly she had a band of babysitters at her disposal. She could be there for her husband yet fret a little less about the care of her young sons.

The thought of asking these women for help had never consciously crossed Randi's mind. Who would expect yoga buddies to be a source of sustenance? But you never know unless you reach out. Sometimes the kindness of strangers makes a huge difference in how you and your mate may cope.

REACHING OUT TO A SUPPORT GROUP

"People call on Sunday night after they've come home from a weekend away or enjoyed other activities. They want Saturdays and Sundays to themselves," comments Angela, an event planner who felt very much on her own as her second husband was being treated for melanoma. "What saved me was a support group for spouses. At least I had something to look forward to. It was also a place where I could vent feelings I couldn't tell him, and feel understood. I could say, 'He's such a baby. He always moans and groans.' If I said that to my friends, they'd think, 'What a bitch. He's got cancer and she only thinks of herself.'"

I've heard similar stories over and over again from women in the midst of their mates' medical crises or involved in long-term caregiving. Life can be lonely and stressful, even if you have the support of friends and family. Much as they may love and help you, they can't truly understand what's it's like for you, because they aren't living it. After they drive home or hang up the phone, they're back to the world of "normal." For many people, like Angela, a good support group can fill the gap. The group puts you in touch with others who are experiencing what you're going through and can help relieve some of the strains you face. It can be a place not only where you can discuss your feelings, but also where you can benefit from practical tips, problem solving, and an exchange of information about doctors, treatments, legal questions, and other concerns.

Face-to-Face Support Groups

Angela found her caregiver group through CancerCare, a national nonprofit organization that provides free professional support services to anyone affected by cancer, including caregivers. Her group of husbands and wives was led by a social worker, who could explain issues under discussion and put information into context to head off any misunderstandings.

Support groups can be particularly useful if you are involved in intense, long-term caregiving. I agree with the view of Sharon B. Shaw, LCSW, CGP, who leads groups and trains support group leaders for the Alzheimer's Association of New York. "People say, 'Where else can I cry?'" she explains. "We believe talking in a group about all of one's feelings—anger, helplessness, hopelessness, anxiety about the future, disappointment in family or friends—helps prevent or at least alleviate isolation, illness, and depression." Many caregivers suffer from depression. A support group can lower that risk.

Online Support Groups

Face-to-face support groups aren't for everyone, for a number of reasons. Groups may not be available in your area, or meeting times may be inconvenient (especially if you're working). You may not be able to leave your mate alone, or you lack transportation. Fortunately, Internet support groups have become an option. You can participate regardless of your schedule or where you live, even if you can't get out of the house. Since online groups usually aren't conducted in real time, you can post messages at your convenience that everyone else can read at theirs. There is time to reflect on what you want to write and what others are saying, and it offers a certain amount of privacy. People are often quicker and more willing to disclose personal information online than in person.

Some phone groups are also available that offer some of the benefits of in-person and online support.

Support That Comes to You

The cardiac support group Mended Hearts, which is affiliated with the American Heart Association, offers another kind of help. Mended Hearts volunteers visit heart disease patients and their families in hospitals and rehabilitation facilities. The volunteers share their own experiences of living with heart disease and put a human face on information about lifestyle changes, treatment, recovery, and other issues.

One wife told me, "Mended Hearts is great, because their volunteers have been where you are. You can ask any question without worrying that it's dumb or foolish. You talk to someone who will listen and get it all out of your system. You also hear someone else say, 'This has been done successfully before.' It's almost better for the caregiver than for the patient."

Mended Hearts volunteers serve as vehicles to connect with people. Some patients and spouses eventually become volunteers themselves and find a full social life through the organization's networking opportunities and events.

FINDING AND EVALUATING
A SUPPORT GROUP

You can find caregiver support groups through hospitals and houses of worship, the organization specific to your mate's condition (such as the American Cancer Society or the American Stroke Association), and the Well Spouse Association, a nonprofit organization that provides support for spouses and partners of the chronically ill and disabled. In disease-specific groups, you're privy to the latest information on the illness. (See the Resources section at the back of this book for contact information.)

When choosing the best group for you, the goal is to match your needs with appropriate support. Here's how:

Know what you want out of the group.

Is it information only? Then you can go to education meetings and learn about legal, financial, and medical issues. Or are you primarily interested in airing and sharing feelings? Most people need both.

Know where you are in the disease process.

Needs differ accordingly, and you want to know whether a particular group will fulfill them. Are you dealing with:

- **A new diagnosis?** You have lots of information and strategic planning needs. If your husband's illness is in the early stage, it may be difficult to be in a group of people whose mates are terminal. At this point, too much information about the future can be overwhelming. You may not want to know everything you'll be up against, even if the disease isn't fatal. There is always a concern about people who are dealing with a new diagnosis entering a group and hearing talk about lack of treatment options or other off-putting information,

■ **Post-treatment issues?** Your partner may be having a hard time getting back to a normal life, including returning to work (or adjusting to not working). Or he may be depressed. You need help with managing your future.

■ **Advanced disease?** You need support and guidance regarding issues like hospice, advance directives, handling your emotions at this tough time, and dealing with life ahead.

■ **Chronic illness?** You may be left feeling burned out from years of caregiving or frightened about what's next. You want to know how others have coped with loneliness, isolation, and other issues involved in long-term care, and need a place to share feelings and thoughts that may seem selfish or shameful.

Ask if prospective members are screened.

This helps assure the best possible "fit" with the group. Some people leave groups complaining that members are "downers," everyone complains, and members' spouses keep dying.

It may also help to find a group as close to your own age group as possible. If you're thirty-five, a group for young adults under forty can help you deal with developmental life issues, such as raising young children with a sick dad. Although groups in that age range can be hard to find, CancerCare does offer them online. On the other hand, some people benefit from participating in a group of varied ages. Words of wisdom can come from unexpected sources.

SIX WAYS TO REACH OUT EFFECTIVELY

YOU MAY BE surprised at how much potential support is readily available. These steps will help you maximize assistance:

1. **Look at the idea of asking for help with new eyes.**

   The Reverend Elizabeth Koffron-Eisen, who runs caregiver support groups for Well Spouse Association, has coined a phrase to describe asking for help. She calls it "double gifting," and explains, "We all know how good we feel when we can help someone. If I have a need and ask for help in a respectful and appreciative way, I give other people the opportunity to help me. And then they have the opportunity to feel good about themselves. They give me a gift, and in turn, I give them a gift." When you find yourself balking at reaching out, Reverend Eisen's philosophy may help.

2. **Try to delegate as much as possible.**

   I often hear people say, "How can I ask my daughter who has toddlers to help? How can I ask my friends, who are sick and tired of hearing my problems?" These are often handy excuses to avoid getting assistance. What's forgotten is the fact that you can't help your man if you're exhausted and become sick yourself. When you can't do everything, you need someone to be a liaison between you and the world. The more specific you can be when delegating, the better—for example, "Fran, can you take Rob to the surgeon's appointment on Friday morning?" or

"Ben, can you help me out with Rob's disability insurance paperwork?" Often friends and family members want to help but don't know how.

3. **Talk to everyone, and welcome surprising bounty.**

You never know who can make a difference. In one case, a men's group at church assembled a contingent to help Claudia, whose husband had Alzheimer's disease. Volunteers took her husband out for a few hours every day. Imagine what a boon this was for Claudia. She was freed to take a nap, balance the checkbook, call friends, or go out herself. Accepting help not only gave her stress-relieving downtime, it also allowed her husband to have valuable experiences with other men.

Think of neighbors who might be interested in sharing resources. One wife was able to share her husband's wheelchair with someone living nearby. Both needed the chair only occasionally. The two never would have known about their matching needs if they hadn't talked with people and said, "I could really use—" or "Do you know anyone who—?" Some people share aides when they don't need (or can't afford) full-time help.

But avoid spilling your deepest thoughts to everyone you meet. Use your judgment. There's a difference between asking for help and baring your soul. If you notice people's eyes glazing over, or if they suddenly have to run to an appointment, ask yourself, "Am I disclosing too much? Am I overdoing it?"

4. **Consider a support group, and choose one wisely.**

There's tremendous comfort in knowing you are not alone and that others are in the same spot. Decide whether you're better off online or with a face-to-face group.

Realize that each option has rules and limits. In a face-to-face group you can't always talk as much as you want, because others need attention, too. You must be willing to listen to their problems and to discussions of issues that may not always concern you. For online groups, you need Internet access and a certain amount of computer savvy, plus a willingness to post and share your thoughts with other people. The more you're willing to put into a group, the more you're likely to get out of it.

When you try a group, give it some time before you decide if it meets your needs. Attend three or more times before making a decision to stay or leave. Often, you can't tell if a group is right for you in one session.

Many groups have a professional leader (or two), such as a social worker, a facilitator, or at least an experienced moderator. This person can put in perspective frightening information or experiences that are discussed and can explain and clarify. A leader also makes sure a few people don't monopolize the time, and that someone's anger toward other members doesn't spiral out of control.

If you're not suited to support groups, you may be better off in individual counseling. Check with your disease-specific organization to see if it offers free counseling. CancerCare and some other organizations do. Or a combination of group and individual therapy may work best for you. See pages 73, 188, 209, and 223–224 for full information on when and how therapy can help.

5. **Recognize that illness brings out the best (and worst) in people.**

Angela, whose friends disappeared on weekends, tells the story of one friend who appeared at her door with prepared food from a gourmet deli. "I thanked her and said, 'Come in,' but she wouldn't." Either this friend thought cancer was catching—a misconception that is more common than we realize—or she felt inadequate or threatened being around someone dealing with desperate illness. Or maybe she didn't want to intrude. We don't know the answer, but the result was that Angela felt angry. "I didn't want food. I needed her company," says Angela.

One of the purposes of this book is to help you verbalize what you need when your mate is ill instead of walking around under a dark cloud. We don't know what would have happened if Angela had said, "I really want your company. Can you find time to visit?" That approach does risk rejection, but it's also possible you may get what you want.

In other cases, you may wish certain people would disappear. Perhaps you have a mother-in-law who criticizes you for not being as attentive to her son as she feels you should be. Have the courage to say something like, "Those comments hurt me and are not helpful at this time."

Conversely, you may discover valuable traits in people. In one situation where a husband was fighting for his life, the couple (understandably) tended to panic and rush to a fatalistic bottom line. They felt so grateful that his father, an elderly physician, was around. His upbeat attitude calmed them down and gave them perspective. His connections in the medical community helped them get immediate appointments with specialists and cut through red tape.

6. Make lists.

At the very time you feel confused and besieged by competing demands, you can make a few key lists to help you find your way through the chaos. Lists impart a sense of control and they calm many people by helping them to focus. They can make responsibilities seem less overwhelming. If lists work for you, start writing. If they make you anxious and you don't know where to start, reach out. Ask a friend, your teenage daughter, or someone else you trust to help you with a list (or make one for you).

Following are two essential lists. Fill out both and review them, especially before holding a family meeting. The lists provide basic information you need to match tasks with people and get help.

WHO CAN I TURN TO? LIST

Fill out this list to identify your own human resources. Put a check mark next to the people, organizations, and programs that can be useful.

FAMILY

☐ His parents   ☐ Children

☐ Your parents   ☐ Stepchildren

☐ His siblings   ☐ Other relatives

☐ Your siblings

FRIENDS

_____

_____

_____

NEIGHBORS

_____

_____

_____

COMMUNITY

☐ Members of your church or other place of worship

☐ Clergy

☐ Volunteer or business groups you belong to

☐ Advocacy and voluntary health organizations, such as the American Cancer Society, American Stroke Association, Alzheimer's Association, or National Family Caregivers Association (which educates and supports caregivers)

☐ Programs such as Meals on Wheels, senior centers, adult day care, or respite care, which gives you a temporary break

WHAT KIND OF HELP DO I NEED? LIST

I need assistance with:

☐ Babysitting

☐ Carpooling

☐ Meal preparation

☐ Finances

☐ Research

☐ Legal matters

☐ Health insurance details

☐ Time off for myself or other family needs

☐ Home maintenance

☐ Shopping

☐ Transportation to hospitals, doctors, therapy sessions, support group meetings

☐ Emotional support

Add to or subtract from this list as necessary. Your needs will differ from someone else's, depending on what's going on, whether care is temporary or long term, whether you have children (and how old they are), whether you're employed, and other factors.

YOU ARE NOT ALONE

IN THE EARLY frontier days, pioneers in this country had to take care of their own. There wasn't any other help around. But times have changed, and that's no longer the case. As the late psychiatrist M. Scott Peck wrote in his book *The Different Drum: Community Making and Peace,* "How strange that we should ordinarily feel compelled to hide our wounds when we are all wounded! Community requires the ability to expose our wounds and weaknesses to our fellow creatures."

There may be times when you feel you are falling apart. At such moments, just remember two words: reach out.

Reflections

🐦 *Seeking or allowing help is a sign of strength.*

🐦 *Help can be all around you. Just open your eyes (and mouth).*

🐦 *Consider a support group.*

🐦 *Delegate, delegate.*

🐦 *Remember—and make use of—the lists in this chapter to match what you need with people who can help.*

5

Keeping the
Family Stable

On a family vacation in San Francisco, your mate stretches out on the hotel bed as your four-year-old daughter jumps on his stomach. Severe gastrointestinal pains follow. Fast-forward many months (and tests) later, and a diagnosis is confirmed. It's cancer. The world as you know it spins off its axis. At the same time that you're reeling, you must help your two children get through what's ahead—and care for him, too.

❧

A mate's chronic illness, such as lung disease or rheumatoid arthritis, has made its impact over time, slowly disrupting family life. Shifts in routine shake up the household and affect the kids. The effort to help him get through his days is sapping your time and energy, while you also have to cope with an agonizing decision to place your mother in a nursing home.

Whatever the scenario, when severe illness strikes your partner, one thing is certain: the event places unexpected demands on everyone. Although the degree and timing of upheaval varies, the challenge is similar: you must stay as stable as you can and function as well as you can. Your mate is also a son and perhaps a sibling. He may have children or grandchildren of his own, and you may have an extended family as well. There are times when you will probably feel inadequate as you juggle responsibilities, especially when everyone else may also be frightened. It's too much to do alone.

HELPING CHILDREN COPE

WHATEVER KIND OF dad your husband may be—fun-loving and affectionate, or distant and removed—he represents security and comfort for the kids. When he is ill, they feel confused and alarmed. The goal is to help them feel as safe and secure as possible and adjust to the changes going on at home. Be present as best you can, and provide information that is appropriate for their age.

"I never lied to my kids. I tried to tell them that they needed to get on with their lives, and they have done that. My husband sees their accomplishments," says Julia, whose mate was paralyzed in an accident during her children's teen years.

Some moms err in telling children too much about Dad's condition. Others say too little, trying to keep kids from worrying too much. They underestimate how seriously children take the medical event or how resilient they will be. A common but mistaken belief is that hiding the facts or pretending a serious diagnosis is minor will protect children. In fact, keeping secrets from kids may lead them to make up their own stories, which can be far worse than the reality.

The goal is to find a balance, and it's a little like the story of "The Three Bears." You want to give kids enough simple facts— not too little, not more than they can absorb, but just enough. It helps to listen for their questions, watch their reactions, and then drip slow and steady information.

Young Children

Young children's fantasies are infinite. They've read graphic literature such as Grimm's fairy tales or Maurice Sendak, and they usually have richer imaginations than adults realize. They may think the worst, confuse the facts, or with utter simplicity skip right to the bottom line: "Is Dad going to lose his leg? Does a heart attack mean his heart is destroyed?" Such honest, direct questions may startle you, and you may feel at a loss for answers. Your task is to explain what is happening in a way your child can understand—and do it together with your mate, if that's possible. It is reassuring if their dad can talk to them in a comforting manner. Choose a time when you're both relaxed, not upset. If he can't participate, ask a calm, caring relative or friend to fill in for him. Or if necessary, take a deep breath and talk with the children yourself.

To begin, it's always helpful to give the illness a name:-"Daddy is sick. Maybe you've heard the word *heart disease*." A label makes the condition real and tangible. Talk about what you'll do about it:"He's going to have an operation to help him." Since his illness will change their lives in some ways, discuss how: "Daddy won't be able to drive you to school in the morning till he's feeling better. Aunt Jean will take you instead." It's reassuring to mention people who will substitute for Dad (or you) in handling some of his responsibilities. Children often worry about who will take care of *them*. When you don't have certain information, say so, but add, "We'll find out." Try to give a realistic yet positive spin.

Answering Questions

Simple language is best in responding to a three-year-old's "Where's Daddy?" An answer might be, "He's in the hospital, and we're all working to get him well." Try to limit answers to the specific questions asked, even though you may feel the urge to elaborate. Remember the "Three Bears rule" when talking with very young children: give them just the amount of information they need. Young children can only digest small amounts of information in one sitting.

I encourage parents of, say, a six-year-old to keep explanations short and simple rather than go into detail, which only confuses and frustrates youngsters. If you say, "Dad had to go to the hospital because he's sick," you can then wait to see which questions follow. This is also a good time to practice your listening skills. Try to pick up on kids' unasked questions; then you can respond with what they really want to know. For example, they may wonder whether they might get sick like Dad. One answer might be: "Anything is possible, but it's doubtful. After all, you are young and healthy, and your body is in good shape." In fact this can be a good time to remind kids to eat well and get enough sleep. At this age and a bit older, kids often wonder if they have done something to make Dad ill. It is helpful to reassure them that his illness is nobody's fault, and certainly not theirs.

Prepare yourself for some challenges, because children have a way of cutting right to the heart of the matter. One mom whose husband had a deadly cancer recalls sitting in the car at a red light when her six-year-old asked, "Is Daddy going to die?" At first she answered "No." The boy kept badgering, "Really—will he?" The third time he repeated the question, she finally replied, "You know, if Daddy dies, we will be okay. We will miss him. We will cry. But we will be okay." She found those words were exactly what he needed. Children's fears can be very raw. When you reassure them at a basic level that life will go on, they are better able to think realistically and positively.

Older Children

The older the children, the more they can know, and the more involved they can be. You can get more detailed with teenagers, but use good judgment. If you tell them, "Dad has multiple sclerosis," don't add a sentence like, "He has to do certain things, because if he doesn't, he may get sick quickly." This sets up the child to worry more about it. The point is, complications may develop down the road, but he isn't going to die tomorrow. You're much better off acknowledging the illness in a realistic way and framing it positively—for example, "If he slows down, eats the right food, and exercises, he should be well for a very long time. However, Dad may need naps more than he used to. If that happens, we can all use this time to go on a picnic or a walk and do things together."

SHOULD CHILDREN VISIT AT THE HOSPITAL?

THE ANSWER DEPENDS on hospital rules and your family's beliefs, of course. If those aren't barriers, I believe kids should see Dad unless they don't want to. (In that case, they can draw something on a card or send a letter instead.) Visiting tends to reduce children's fears and helps them understand that hospitals are places where people can get well. If recovery isn't possible, at least they've seen their father and been exposed to the cycle of life. Illness and death are natural parts of life that children should know about. Try not to be too overprotective.

On the other hand, be ready to talk about the visit in advance, and let kids know what to expect. Hospitals can be strange, intimidating places where Dad may be surrounded by tubes and beeping equipment. To prepare youngsters, consider reading them one of the many children's books available on the topic of a hospitalized parent. Ask your librarian or a knowledgeable bookstore employee to recommend age-appropriate titles.

A common question is "Why did Dad get sick?" An answer might be "We don't know yet. We're working to get him better." If there's a high risk he won't improve, you can add, "We can't promise he will, but we are doing everything possible." It's best to tell the truth, but the truth can be tempered with hope. Since older children understand the concept of death, they may become frightened that Dad could die, and so could you and they.

SOMETIMES AN illness is so sudden, you have no time to prepare your children. You may not be in shape to do more than put one foot in front of the other. In such cases, you may want to ask a friend or relative to take the kids for a few hours (or even overnight) to give you a break. But there is also benefit in circling the wagons. You are still a family unit, and you need the kids as much as they need you. You may feel more comfortable keeping them close to you.

BUILDING
A FAMILY TEAM

WHEN YOUR CHILDREN are old enough to be verbal, you can talk together every day about what's going on. If you're too pressed for time to manage that, try a weekly meeting. You can use this opportunity to catch up with children's activities, such as class trips and projects and news of their friends. Dad's progress (or lack of it) and their feelings about it can be part of the discussion. If young children have little patience for conversation, the meeting can be a good time for a creative activity such as drawing. Kids often express fear and other emotions this way.

Teens may not want to sit down to talk with you, either, but this is one time for firmness. It's best not to let them wriggle out of this designated family time. When her husband was in the hospital with a broken pelvis and its complications, a working mom scheduled a conversation with her twelve- and sixteen-year-old sons on Friday evenings. The twelve-year-old was willing; the sixteen-year-old wanted to be with his friends on the weekend and didn't want to talk. She offered this compromise: "You must have this time with me. Tell me what other day of the week would make it easier for you." She gave him a choice and got something in return. He picked Tuesday.

This is the same technique that works with defiant young children. When you tell a child, "Get in the car," you set up opportunities for opposition that lead to temper tantrums. Offer a choice instead, such as "Would you like to ride in the back or the front seat?" The choice empowers the child, which can diffuse a potentially explosive situation. You can use this approach in other ways when Dad is ill. You might ask, "Would you like to visit Dad today or tomorrow?" or "Would you like Grandma to stay with you on Monday or Tuesday?" These questions set up a limited parameter that reduces the possibility of "no."

WATCH YOUR EMOTIONS IN FRONT OF CHILDREN

THERE'S A fine line between inviting young children into the experience of their father's illness and overwhelming them with your own anxiety. If your mate suffers one setback after another and you can't stand it anymore, by all means go into the bathroom, cry your heart out, or scream in the shower. If you have to, throw up. Just don't do it in front of the kids. Small children especially need a stable force in their lives.

That doesn't mean that you can't ever let the kids see you feeling sad or shedding tears. After all, you may be bombarded at times with feelings of despair, fear, and anxiety. The issue is taking care not to lose control and make them more frightened than they may already be. They need your strength. Lend as much of yours as you can.

Dealing with Children's Reactions

Children may react in any number of ways when Dad is sick. Because young children may not verbalize their feelings, signs of upset come out in other ways, such as crying or fighting with friends. Watch behavior for cues. They may withdraw or become clingy, have nightmares, stop eating or overeat, or become depressed. Child and adolescent depression looks different at different ages. In a ten- or twelve-year-old it may be expressed with irritability and refusal to do homework or chores around the house. It's common for a child who doesn't speak out to act out instead. A fifteen- or sixteen-year-old may be more vocal and rebellious. A child who is struggling with a parent's health status may suffer a decline in school performance or lose interest in basketball practice or spending time with friends or even turn to drugs or alcohol.

The most disturbing reaction from children that you may have to deal with is anger. Because kids feel scared and often don't know how to talk about their fears, they may lash out instead. Think of how often you may have wanted to blame someone for not taking good enough care of you. Children feel that way, too. Here you are trying to do your best, and your teenage daughter rolls her eyes and gives you a look that says you're not very smart. In cases where the impact of illness happens gradually, a child may have adjustment problems over time rather than immediately.

Regardless of the situation, trust yourself to know your child. "When you sense something is different, something is different," advises Kathleen McCue, MA, CCLS, in her book *How to Help Children Through a Parent's Serious Illness.*

DEALING WITH
THE REST OF THE FAMILY

RELATIONSHIPS WITH RELATIVES—both his and yours—are fundamental to family stability when your husband is seriously ill. Some families have never been close, but when illness occurs, all of your relatives tend to be affected. This event is an assault on the family structure. A crisis suddenly reminds cousins, aunts and uncles, and the brother-in-law you always fought with that invisible bonds connect them. Sometimes the illness can be an opportunity to heal relationships and provide a supply of helpers. At other times it may bring only unwanted stress. When you're feeling under siege, the challenge is to rise to your best self.

Unexpected Positive Changes

When you accept that all families are imperfect (not just yours), positive experiences often follow. I remember a friend of mine, Sally, who attended a family funeral while her husband lay recovering from a second heart attack. She told me:

I hadn't been close to my husband's siblings and their spouses, but I found myself feeling so happy to be with them at this difficult time. I felt such a sense of belonging and connection, as we sat side by side at the service, went to the cemetery, and then shared a meal. We were family, as flawed as our unit was. It changed my whole attitude toward my husband's family.

From then on, I made a real effort to stay in touch. I also never realized that one of my brothers-in-law would become such an asset. He came to the hospital almost every day, sat with me, and because he was so easy to be with, he became an

*enormous comfort. I felt I could call at three a.m. if I had to,
and he would come running if I needed him. I'm very lucky.*

Another woman tried to find common ground with her sister-in-law. She discovered they both loved the same novels and shared the same taste in fashion. They had fun shopping together. Your relatives don't have to be your closest buddies, but perhaps they can fill a valuable niche as well-meaning people who add to your life.

BLENDED FAMILIES

BECAUSE FAMILIES CAN be complicated today, you may be in a second or third marriage, where your family group includes more than one set of in-laws. Or yours may be a blended family, where you may have to deal with his children. If young stepchildren visit only part time, their routine may be disrupted when their father is sick. They may feel so frightened that they take it out on the most available target—you—and their words may sting. You may have to swallow your pride and ask his ex or a member of his family to help with his children.

His children may blame you for their dad's illness, finding all kinds of irrational reasons why you're at fault, such as, "You should have made him exercise." It may be up to you to reach out to them. It's totally unfair on top of everything else you have to do, but it's reality.

Healing Rifts

Because everyone is on edge at a time like this, conflicts can arise with your mate's children or other relatives even when they try to be useful. In one instance, a husband had just come home from the hospital after quadruple bypass surgery. His wife,

Rosemary, was consumed with worry about him. Of course, his children (her stepchildren) wanted to be there to help. His twenty-five-year-old daughter took charge of the laundry—a seemingly simple and generous gesture. When she removed the load from the dryer, however, she folded the sheets her way—the wrong way in Rosemary's view. Stressed out with fear for her husband, Rosemary exploded like a popping pressure cooker—a reaction that was totally out of character for her. Hurt feelings and arguments ensued.

It took months for family healing to begin, and unfortunately scars still exist; Rosemary and her stepdaughter still have a way to go. The reality is, when you feel panicked and overwhelmed, you lack your usual patience. Sometimes a fight can be diffused immediately with an apology: "I'm sorry I blew up at you." In other cases, it takes a long stretch to work out enmity between you. But that doesn't mean bad feelings can't ultimately be handled.

Mistakes are why pencils have erasers and computers have a "delete" key. It is never too late to try to explain or apologize. In my own life, days or weeks after an angry exchange (yes, even professionals mess up at times) I tell people, "You know, I've been thinking about what happened, and . . ." Often it surprises the other person that you, too, have been concerned about the rift and that it pains you just as much as it does them.

Nothing is perfect. You do the best you can. In times of crisis, sometimes people do lose their tempers, slam doors, and cry.

Be Prepared for Disappointments

There are times when the problem is family distance rather than disagreement. One set of in-laws never visited their son in all his months of being treated for colon cancer. "His parents deal with problems by sticking their heads in the sand. They called, but didn't see him in person," says Myra.

Other people discover their *own* parents won't be there for them. A client I worked with, just married for the second time, felt shell-shocked as her new husband lay in intensive care after an industrial accident. Her confidence fled, and she realized that she desperately wanted her parents' support—a common reaction. When she asked them to fly in from another state to spend a few weeks with her, they refused. In therapy she finally acknowledged that they had repeatedly let her down throughout her life. Their lack of support brought back many painful wishes from childhood, such as, "If only my parents could be different."

Even the strongest caregiver has a piece of her that wants to be taken care of. Fortunately, although this woman's own parents were not supportive, her in-laws showed up in force. They helped her with hospital visits and all the sitter services she required.

SIX WAYS TO KEEP YOUR FAMILY UNIT STRONG

IT CAN TAKE all the patience and energy you possess to nurture and coordinate your own nuclear household and keep it steady. Then you also have to cope with extended family. Here's how to do your best:

1. **Make time to be a mother.**

    Your kids need your attention, no matter how busy you are. When you're so involved in coping with your partner and his situation, you may lose sight of the fact that the children are trying to cope, too. They need your attention and affection, as well as routines.

    Regular schedules reassure children and make them feel safe. That doesn't mean there won't have to be disruptions.

Nothing is perfect, and this may be a rough time, but you can minimize changes. Someone else may be able to pinch-hit for you at the hospital for a while or accompany your mate to a test, allowing you to focus on the kids.

Every Tuesday, a grandfather spent the entire day at the bedside of his son-in-law, a cancer patient, freeing his daughter from this duty. "That one day a week I could just be 'Bobby's mother.' It was so important that my poor kid had one normal day with his mom available," she says.

Another mom, Brenda, dropped her daughter off at school every day. She worked from nine to three and then headed for the hospital. A friend agreed to pick up the kids at the end of the school day. Brenda and her child spent time together every morning and shared dinner at night.

2. **Look for ways children can help.**

Allow children to feel there is something they can contribute. A four-year-old can make a picture for Daddy. You can ask teenagers to cook dinner, do the dishes, make phone calls for you, or (if they can drive) chauffeur younger children to school. Just don't overdo the task load.

All of you gain strength by working together as a team. If everyone communicates, the longer the illness goes on, the more you can lean on one another. Remember, you're a family unit. Try to have meals together as often as possible to reinforce feelings of connection.

3. **Focus on the positives of extended family.**

Relatives are part of the family stabilization system. Take advantage of their strengths, and concentrate on how they can help rather than on past hurts. Some families nurse grievances for decades, but there are times in life when individual family dynamics must give way to the immediate greater good. Forgiveness works better than blame.

Illness is a time to focus on what's really important in life. If you can give up your grudge and try to find common ground, you may have a helpful new resource. You will be the one who benefits.

Sometimes you just have to become more tolerant if you need help. And of course, learn to hold close those helpers who are dear. If your stepson is a good mechanic, put him in charge of your car maintenance and tell him how much you appreciate him.

4. **Say no to people who are "energy takers."**

There are so many benefits when you can work together with family. However, if that's not your experience, try to remember that your mate's illness frightens everyone. Fear can generate tension as old patterns of interaction are reintroduced. Just because you may be willing to forgive and forget, it doesn't mean all others will do the same. If your mother-in-law still prefers to hold on to her anger, you may have no choice but to stay away. You have to be able to set limits and say no to "energy takers." Surround yourself with "energy givers" instead.

Other people may mean well yet mindlessly meddle or try to tell you what to do. There are those who constantly bombard you with stories of others they know and methods that helped them. "Did you try acupuncture (or vitamin C)?" they ask. When you don't want to hear this information, change the subject. If that doesn't work, you may have to say something like, "I appreciate your concern, but this advice isn't useful to me right now." Or designate someone else to deal with the person.

5. **Consider professional help for your family.**

   Any management of a chronic disease is a burden on the family. It isn't necessarily the diagnosis that hits spouses and children as much as the ongoing mainte- nance. For example, if Dad has diabetes, it's often helpful when someone monitors how the family is doing psycho- logically and emotionally. Sometimes you can take advantage of mental health services associated with a dia- betes clinic. Some people think it will make things worse if they go to family counseling and talk about issues, but the opposite may be true.

   A few hospitals, such as the Cleveland Clinic, offer ongoing services for children who have a very sick par- ent. The school guidance counselor, nurse, or your child's teacher can be helpful when your child seems to be hav- ing problems, especially if you let those people know in advance what's going on. If you have privacy concerns, you have every right to insist on confidentiality. The child's pediatrician or family doctor can be helpful, too.

   Check out resources for families offered by the organ- ization for your mate's disease. For example, the American Cancer Society provides information online and in print on talking with children about a parent's cancer. CancerCare for Kids provides fact sheets on how to help a child cope with a parent's illness—plus free online, phone, and face-to-face counseling for children and for parents.

6. **Remember, you and your husband have the final say.**

   Your husband's family may have different value sys- tems from yours and readily voice their opinions.

Feelings can run high in a medical crisis, and sometimes well-meaning relatives may differ among themselves on the best course to get him well. Some may push for aggressive treatment, while others feel differently. It isn't easy to cope with everyone's needs and input. The bottom line is that the decision rests with the patient and his wife. If he can't participate, and treatment decisions must be made quickly, you as the spouse are the final arbiter. If you are an unmarried partner, a health care proxy that names you to make health care decisions in accordance with your partner's wishes can help head off arguments with his family.

In cases where there is disagreement with his relatives, the best thing you can do is invite them to a family meeting. It may be helpful to bring in a family therapist or a member of the clergy to such a meeting to help reduce tension and friction. If his family doesn't accept your invitation, at least you offered it.

KEEPING THE FAMILY AFLOAT

WHEN YOUR MATE is seriously ill, life is a stormy sea for everyone. His battle has an immediate impact on the family, and it threatens the future. That's a good reason to make sure your children don't get lost in the shuffle of everything else you have to do. At the very time you need them to behave, kids can be sensitive to change and need you more than ever. If you and your youngster are going through a bad patch, you can always suggest that the child talk to a family member or even a friend's understanding parent. The point is for the child to express feelings to a caring, knowledgeable adult.

We now live in a society where families are splintered, but a major event like serious illness usually touches all family members and sometimes draws them together. At its best, family is a source of both help and sanctuary. However, remember that you are the center of stability. To stay strong, try to increase your flexibility. As one wife observes, "It's amazing how loose you can become. It's brittleness and perfectionism that kill you." Amen.

Reflections

- *Understand that your kids are trying to cope with Dad's illness, too.*

- *Try to give children just enough information.*

- *Work as a team with relatives if you can—both his and yours.*

- *Realize that it helps to forgive.*

- *You're the spouse; you have the final say.*

PART TWO

Taking Care
of Him

6

Understanding
Your Man

Do you recognize your mate in any of the scenarios below? Check all that apply:

☐ He complains about pain yet won't take the medication that relieves it.

☐ He refuses to exercise, eat right, or lose weight despite the doctor's warnings that his lifestyle could kill him.

☐ He showers praise on the home care nurse, when you're the one who's up all night with him.

☐ He picks fights with the children.

☐ He wants you available 24/7, when his condition doesn't warrant it.

☐ He snaps and criticizes everything you do.

☐ He chatters endlessly, saying nothing that matters.

☐ He refuses to get out of bed for days (or weeks) on end.

☐ He withdraws and won't tell you how he feels.

☐ He ignores worrisome symptoms, refusing to call the doctor.

☐ He won't allow others to help you care for him.

☐ He thinks he has a new disease every day.

☐ He denies that anything is wrong.

☐ He whines and whines.

If you've checked three or more of these statements, you're in good company. This is just a partial list of comments I've heard from women who are taking care of sick partners. Puzzled and frustrated, they often ask me, "Why does he behave that way?" I smile with empathy and tell them that anyone in a relationship knows men and women are truly different. Then I help them understand how those differences play out during a man's illness. Men do not always behave in useful ways when they're sick. If you realize that he's just being a guy, and try to understand your differences, his actions make more sense. It's easier to manage your own anger or annoyance at him and focus on the goal: helping him when he needs you so much.

OUR MACHO CULTURE AND YOUR PARTNER'S HEALTH

OF COURSE IT drives you crazy if your mate ignores pain controlling (and even lifesaving) medical advice or alarming symptoms that would send you dashing to the doctor. It's tough enough to take care of him without also fighting his resistance to getting help. Consider this harrowing experience related by a woman I'll call Caroline. When her husband was diagnosed with prostate cancer, the couple flew to a major medical center in Los Angeles for surgery. Although the operation went well, he had lots of healing to do. He promised Caroline that on the trip back home he would go through the long airport corridors sitting in a wheelchair. "When the time came, the airport was mobbed, and there he was, hooked up to a catheter," Caroline recalls. "Then he suddenly decided he didn't need a wheelchair. He felt it was 'unmanly.' I told him, 'It is not unmanly. Nobody cares,' but he wouldn't listen. He had trouble walking; he worried that the catheter would fall out. I had to scurry around him like a little terrier to prevent people from jostling him. It had to be the worst afternoon of my life."

Although it may be hard to imagine thinking, "Wheelchairs are for sissies," that attitude is fairly common among men. It may breed reckless behavior that could set him back or impede his recovery. This behavior becomes easier to understand when you look at its origins. Male attitudes toward health care trace back to "tough guy" lessons learned in boyhood.

"Our culture has taught men that they should stifle their pains, deny their symptoms, and wait as long as possible before visiting a doctor," says Robert N. Butler, MD, president of the International Longevity Center. He adds that many men consider it unmanly to maintain a regular relationship with their doctor.

Although men have been given permission to be more sensitive today, too few break free of the message to "suck it up." Some men will ignore the symptoms of a heart attack until they actually collapse and someone else has to rush them to the emergency room. I know of a husband who went even further: he refused to go to the hospital despite chest pains. He died at home early the next morning .

Men also tend to think they're invincible until something happens. They're less likely to get checkups, perform self-exams for conditions like testicular cancer, or take other preventive health measures. When they do become ill, they're less likely to follow their doctor's orders. "No lifting," a physician warns a man recovering from abdominal surgery. Yet two days later the patient picks up a heavy bag. "It's okay. I can do it," he assures his partner. Another man tries to drive his car two weeks after a major heart attack, ignoring orders for complete rest. His wife has to hide the keys.

Is it any wonder, then, that men die on average five years earlier than women? That's an improvement over the seven-year gap back in 1990. Yet men still have higher fatality rates than women for all leading causes of death, including heart disease and lung cancer. Despite this reality (and although he may go to the gym and want to *look* great), the average American male still doesn't put much effort into his physical or mental well-being. It's enough to make you throw up your hands and surrender, but one of your jobs is to protect your partner from himself. You're not always as helpless as you may feel.

ILLNESS FALLOUT:
YOUR MATE'S ANGER AND NEEDINESS

WHEN YOUR PARTNER is sick, he feels weak and out of control, which probably doesn't fit his masculine image. He may respond with childish behavior or lash out at the handiest targets—you and possibly your children, if you have them. In addition, he may feel threatened by the fact that you're in charge and by the enforced intimacy involved in receiving personal care. He may bark at, bait, or criticize you, and withdraw instead of facing his feelings of helplessness. Although it is true that some men are more attuned to their emotions these days, many still are not.

In his book *When Good Men Behave Badly,* David B. Wexler, PhD, a clinical psychologist, describes his behavior toward his wife when severe back pain sent him to bed for several weeks. "The pain was the least of it; the dependency was the killer. I couldn't stand needing her so much. Her helping me was like a broken mirror reminding me of my inadequate state, and I acted nastier and nastier to her."

DOES YOUR PARTNER'S NEEDINESS THREATEN YOU?

SOME WOMEN call their men "big babies" and complain, "He could never survive pregnancy and childbirth." If you find yourself feeling this way, pay attention to your response to his neediness. Does it threaten you because it deviates from your male ideal? Do you also buy into the myth that a real man is strong all the time? I've worked with many women who cringe at their mate's vulnerability or complaints. Some feel frightened that their rock is no longer solid, especially if he starts to cry, as some men do. Although you may view his tears as "acting like a baby," he really needs you—along with a loving hug.

This is a time to reexamine your definition of "masculinity." Is it based on a fantasy of physical strength, emotional control, and power? Some women pay lip service to wanting sensitive men but don't cope well with their sensitive behavior. If you truly don't know what to do with his emotions, walk away and take a breath, then come back. Remember how you felt when you faced loss—how much you needed his arms around you. Even if you can't hug him, reach out and touch his shoulder so that he knows you're still there.

One wife used to panic when her husband broke down and cried in despair. "I no longer do that," she observes. "I've learned he does pull out of it. It doesn't last forever. I've also come to realize I don't have to fix it for him. I'm able to listen calmly and just be there. That's what he needs."

Such behavior really doesn't have anything to do with you, although your partner's words and conduct toward you hurt just the same. In return for your warmth and caring, he berates you. You do need to vent, but not at him—not while he's down. If you think he can hear you, tell him, "Please stop. I'm trying to help you." If he doesn't hear you, you may have to bite your lip to avoid a fight. Research shows that upset, nagging, and hostility can interfere with his recovery. Even small spats can inhibit the immune system and impede healing.

That said, you don't have to be a candidate for sainthood. You need somewhere else to blow off steam. A support group of others in your position or a trusted friend can help you cope when it's a stretch to tolerate his behavior and it is just too much for you to deal with. Remember, your job is to be a valuable helpmate, maintain compassion, and avoid becoming bitter and resentful.

EXAGGERATED PERSONALITY TRAITS

ANOTHER REASON A seriously sick man may be difficult for you to handle is that illness tends to exaggerate personality traits. There you are, upset to begin with—often worrying about life-and-death issues—and on top of it all you must cope with irritating personality changes in your mate. In those moments you may not feel loving at all. Understanding what to expect can help.

For example, you may be married to a Type A man who is accustomed to ordering a staff of employees around. His lack of control when he's sick may cause him (consciously or unconsciously) to assert himself, acting like he's the general and you're the troops. His litany of "Do this . . . do that . . . why did you—" may be more than your fraying patience can stand.

If your man is an extrovert, he may babble endlessly as a way of coping. Senseless talking keeps him from facing what's happening.

Or instead of resting when he should, he may engage in confusing, senseless running around. This may be just an exaggerated version of his usual coping style.

Or maybe he's the strong, silent type. He may grow even quieter when he's ill, and he probably won't tell you what he needs, what he wants, or especially what he feels in a direct manner. Instead of admitting he's terrified of going to the hospital, he may refuse to report alarming shortness of breath to the doctor (and forbid you to do so). When women are anxious or afraid, they tend to let people in more easily than men do. They feel better after they discuss facts and feelings with others. Many men react differently.

"Going it alone had been my badge of honor. How foolish. I confused silence with strength. I have come to see that as the classic male mistake," writes the journalist and former award-winning television producer Richard M. Cohen in his best-selling book, *Blindsided: Lifting a Life Above Illness: A Reluctant Memoir.* Cohen, who is married to the TV journalist Meredith Vieira, with whom he has three children, recounts his long struggle with multiple sclerosis and two successfully treated bouts of colon cancer—and as a result, his redefinition of what it is to be a strong man.

IS YOUR PARTNER DEPRESSED?

DEPRESSION, WHICH OFTEN goes hand in hand with illness, may be a factor in his difficult behavior and is often triggered by his condition or the pain involved. As many as one-third of seriously ill patients have symptoms of depression, according to the Cleveland Clinic. Depression is especially likely to occur in cases of heart attack, Parkinson's disease, multiple sclerosis, stroke, cancer, and Type 2 diabetes. In fact, any chronic disease raises the risk of depression. Complications and setbacks in a condition can erode confidence and also set off depression.

SYMPTOMS OF DEPRESSION

STAY ALERT to these signs in your man:

- Persistent sadness, restlessness, anxiety, or "empty" mood
- Feelings of hopelessness or pessimism
- Feelings of guilt, worthlessness, or helplessness
- Loss of interest in pleasurable hobbies and activities, including sex
- Fatigue
- Difficulty concentrating or making decisions
- Sleep problems
- Changes in appetite and/or weight
- Suicidal thoughts
- Irritability

Note that depression may be the reason he's aggressive, drinking, drugging, or isn't taking his medications. Men are not only more likely to deny illness, they also are more likely to use recreational drugs and alcohol to numb their feelings.

Nick, a marketing manager, crawled into bed and stayed there for six months after a colostomy. He couldn't cope with the idea of depending on an ostomy bag. Other men become hypochondriacs when they get sick. Instead of realizing that they may be depressed, they think every ache and pain means a life-threatening illness. Underneath, they're really miserable and angry.

Male patients may also get depressed when they lose their usual routines and diversions. It's realistic to feel deep sadness if active sports have always played a significant role in his life and he can no longer jog or play racquetball because of progressive losses from arthritis. If he can't function in the world as he used to, it's another loss. One woman found her mate sitting in the living room sobbing, "What good am I? Nobody needs me. They're handling everything at the office without me."

It's a rare man who is so secure that his self-esteem remains intact when his identity as a breadwinner and his external structure is stripped away. That structure helps define him; without it he may feel adrift. This is a time for understanding. But the task is to get him help, not drown in depression alongside him.

MEDICATIONS CAN CAUSE MOOD CHANGES

BE AWARE THAT certain medications can also affect mood and cause behavioral changes—with sometimes bizarre results. One committed partner was warned to watch for evidence of manic behavior when her husband was treated with the drug prednisone for months. "Some patients go on huge spending sprees," the doctor advised her. Certain drugs used to treat Parkinson's disease (known as dopamine agonists) have been linked with compulsive gambling and even sex addiction.

Hormone treatment for some prostate cancer patients may affect personality. Says a partner who lived through it, "Sometimes I thought he was developing major depression; other times I was convinced he was going bipolar on me. This normally cheerful, capable person temporarily resembled a woman with bad PMS or menopausal symptoms. He had severe hot flashes and developed hair-trigger anger. I knew it was primarily the hormone therapy plus the 'hit' of a cancer recurrence."

It's up to you to follow your mate's mood changes closely and report them to the doctor. There may be alternative drugs he can take, or perhaps dosage can be reduced.

NINE WAYS TO HELP YOUR PARTNER EMOTIONALLY

WHATEVER IS GOING on, the goal is to encourage your mate to become as self-sufficient as possible, help him to gain a sense of control and to feel he has some power—and preserve your own sanity. Here are some ways to accomplish that:

1. **Encourage productive activity.**

   Stop and ask yourself, "What has been taken away from him, and what needs to be replaced?" Many men cope with tension by exercising, walking, or being physically active in other ways. Yet serious illness often eliminates these outlets. Maybe he can try a gentler activity, like yoga, or a meditative martial art, such as tai chi. If he's a gardener who can no longer kneel to plant and weed, perhaps he can use a long-handled tool—or pick berries or clip hedges.

   Or if those options are not possible, are there activities he *can* handle? Encourage him to read or to listen to audio books from the library. Be inventive. If he's a fisherman, get him an illustrated book on the sport. Try to remind him that there's a life out there and activities he enjoys and may be able to return to. If he doesn't respond positively, stop.

   Use whatever resources are available. Perhaps he can solve crossword puzzles, listen to music, play chess or checkers, or even take an art course (online or in person, depending on his condition). One wife often plays video games with her wheelchair-bound husband. He can't walk, but he can participate in activities that engage his mind. Hopefully, the more your partner has to do, the easier he'll be to live with.

Don't let unlimited TV time take over his life and yours. On days when you feel ready to scream, in order to quell your own anxiety you may be tempted to sit him in front of the screen like a child. Yet if he becomes a couch potato, in the long run it does neither of you any good. Television can be a good distraction, but watching it all the time drowns out your shared life and dulls the senses. It can lead him to forget he has other interests and it discourages face-to-face communication.

2. Call his friends.

Men tend to bond over functions like sports and business, but they don't participate in such activities when they're in the hospital or ill at home, where access to male companionship is limited. A man who has few friends outside of sports or work may depend more on you for company. For both your sakes, it's important to help him maintain a social network.

Encourage your partner's guy friends (who often don't know what to do when a buddy is sick) to come over and visit. Let his Tuesday night poker group or his tennis partners know he's interested in company. You can say, "Jack is sick and would love to see you." You can even call their wives, who will suggest that seeing your guy is a good thing to do. Of course, you don't want to overwhelm him with visitors if he's *very* ill. Become the gatekeeper and guardian. Tell people, "Call before you come, just in case he's having a bad afternoon."

A brother-in-law or cousin he likes or his own siblings may be able to help. Don't be afraid to tell them they are like a band of brothers and that family counts. Maybe they can watch the ball game together or even take your mate to a sports event or concert. Special seating is available for the disabled.

It helps if he is active in his place of worship. Men are more likely to rely on friends made through religion-related activities, and that may reduce the pressure on you. Small communities also tend to offer more immediate social support than big cities. People are likelier to know one another and pull together.

If your mate has dementia or Alzheimer's disease, the social isolation can be devastating. Take the initiative to contact family and friends and explain that although the disease has changed your lives, you still value their friendship and support. Consider inviting a few friends or family members over. Let them know in advance of any physical or emotional changes they should be prepared for. Not everyone will respond to your invitation, but some people may surprise you, especially if you suggest ways they can communicate with him and activities they might do together. You never know unless you try.

Remember, if he has his own social circle, he doesn't have to rely so much on you—and it's healthy for him as well. Research shows that men who have a support system live longer.

3. Reassure and comfort him.

If he's seriously ill, he's undoubtedly afraid, whether or not he talks about it. He needs steady doses of affection and healing hope. One man surprised his wife when he suddenly paused from sipping his coffee at breakfast one morning to ask, "Do you think I'll be all right?" He had developed a blood clot in one of his legs for the third time. His wife responded in the only way she knew how: "There's no doubt in my mind that you will be okay. I know in my heart the blood clots will stop, although I don't know when." She felt this was true. Although there was no scientific evidence to support her statement, her words gave him solace. Eventually, a combination of medication and an implanted filter that prevented clots from traveling elsewhere in the body did work for him.

Another spouse found her husband sitting on the sofa with tears running down his face. Shifting into a gentle interrogation mode, she asked, "Is it *this* bothering you? Is it *that*?" He answered that he was fine, but he clearly wasn't fine. "You have to probe it out of men," she says. "Sometimes you really don't feel like doing that, but I did. I finally realized he was overwhelmed by the thought of having cancer. He couldn't handle it. So I kept telling him everything would be all right in a really positive voice. He asked, 'Are you sure?' and I thought to myself, 'What do I know?' But I said yes with ringing authority. I surprised myself. I didn't know what to do, and that answer came to me."

She feels he needed to hear that from her, and it helped her, too. "I didn't really believe it at first, but I found repeating it began to convince me. So far, it *is* all right," she says.

When another husband worried about surviving, his wife, Carla, used her own approach. Sensing that he was dwelling on death, she assured him, "I will always be with you, no matter what. You will never be alone." His body language immediately changed and he relaxed. He went back to reading the newspaper.

Just sitting quietly and holding your mate's hand or putting your arm around him can also be a tremendous comfort to him. It's natural for him to feel unlovable when he's sick and guilty that he's a burden. The actor Michael J. Fox openly expressed some of the unspoken thoughts that tortured him about his marriage to Tracy

Pollan as he was learning to cope with his diagnosis of Parkinson's disease. He said, "There were all these questions that I was really afraid to ask . . . like: Is this not what you bought into? Does it scare you that I'm sick? Do you not want to be with me because I'm sick? Do you not love me because I'm sick?"

Your mate may even say things like, "You'll be better off without me" or "Are you sure you don't want to leave?" Such questions arise when he feels he can't give you what he used to, or that he is not a good father to the children. Yet the last thing he wants is to lose you. In this case, try to decipher the double message. Ignore the words, put them in the trash can, and pay attention to the second, hidden message—"I need your love." A simple statement like, "Of course I won't leave. I love you," makes a huge difference.

Another husband kept telling his wife about his million-dollar life insurance policy, saying, "If I die, you'll get it all and be rich." Somehow she was able to reach into her heart for the ideal response: "There isn't enough money in the world to replace you." He never mentioned it again. Almost every couple I've treated has experienced some version of these dialogues.

4. Encourage resilience.

Ultimately, he'll never get through his illness and its effects on your life together unless he learns to cope with his condition, whatever it is, and finds ways to distract and soothe himself. You can't do it for him, but you can gently nudge him toward this objective. Realize that there's a fine line between empathy and compassion for him and fueling his dependence, denial, or depression. Healthy love and smothering love are not the same; the former enriches, the latter suffocates. Ask yourself, "Am

I monitoring him out of my own anxiety or for his welfare? Does he really need constant care, or is it me who needs to give it?" Some women have a need to help whether it's productive or not.

Conversely, many men expect you to be there all the time, even when it isn't necessary or desirable. If he won't allow anyone else to take care of him so that you can take a break, insist calmly, "I need the help. If I don't get some time to myself, I won't have the strength to be here for you." If you're on edge or feel too resentful to speak quietly, go to another room or take a walk before you tackle the issue. Remember, you're entitled to nurture yourself and have time out. It's important to discuss such issues together. You don't want different expectations to create distance between you.

5. Look beneath the surface.

If he's constantly in conflict with the children, the underlying dynamics may be jealousy or envy. I remember a client who felt so miserable that he envied his kids for the fun they were having. Their antics represented life, and he was afraid he was dying. As a result, every little noise bothered him. He screamed at the children all the time, and he didn't like himself for it.

There are ways to help a man in this spot. He's harnessing all of his energy to get well and has no patience. He can't take much chaos. Children's shrieks do grate on him. Tell the kids, "Daddy is sick. Play outside." Or perhaps a neighbor's house can become their temporary haven. Often, young children have to be kept away.

Meanwhile, reassure your partner that he is still number one, but that realistically you do have to take care of the family, too. He may look at his son, who is dating and beginning a life filled with possibility, and sit there feeling his own future drain away. If your intuition tells you that's what he's feeling, say the words. Tell him, "Remember, hon, when we too thought that life was an endless adventure?"

He also has to know that admitting pain and expressing emotions don't diminish him and are natural human behaviors. You can gently remind him of that by bringing home a book by the poet and writer Robert Bly or other popular authors who encourage men to feel. Just leave it next to him and perhaps suggest in passing that he might find it helpful. Or you can even leave this book within easy reach.

6. Let him take control.

Sometimes your mate's control issues may cause him to balk at the doctor's orders. One wife asked her husband to take walks down the hall in the hospital, as the doctor prescribed. He refused. Then he growled during discharge when she wrote down complicated medication instructions from his doctor. This wife recalls, "I was so mad at him. Then it all became clear to me a day or two later when he blurted out, 'Everyone is telling me what to do.'"

He may need to feel that he's making the decisions. If you choose your words carefully, it can make all the difference. For example, he's likelier to take that walk down the hospital corridor if you say, "What do you think about a walk?" rather than, "You have to get up and walk." Touch his arm or cheek lovingly to help him feel cared for rather than besieged.

If your husband is a diabetic who resists taking care of himself or someone with high blood pressure who won't take his medication regularly, you may feel that you're dealing with an adolescent. Neither nagging nor criticism works, however, even if what he's doing is destructive.

He'll just dig in his heels. Instead of accusing your mate, which makes his behavior the issue, take a different approach. Try something like, "I don't go through what you do during the day, but everything that happens to you does affect me and the whole family. I'm concerned about how you're doing, and I want to know if there's some way I can be more helpful."

When you start a sentence with the word "I," you take ownership of your own needs. That helps to ensure that he won't feel attacked. I advise clients to facilitate discussion in a way that helps their partner to identify his needs, articulate them, and focus on how to meet them.

Remember, too, that what your partner experiences emotionally can vary, depending on the illness. Organizations such as the Arthritis Foundation, the American Cancer Society, or the American Stroke Association can help you understand what's going on and offer tips on how to support him more effectively. Counselors may be available to talk to you.

7. Know when to speak up or stand up to him.

Sometimes nothing works, and you simply have to cave in. At other times you owe it to yourself to speak up. As one doctor advised a wife, "You're going to have to learn to say no to him. He's angry at himself for being helpless." For example, is your partner entitled to home care rehabilitation services that he would rather turn down? Do you believe such services are important and can help him? Explain calmly that he needs the help whether he thinks so or not. If possible, point out a concrete benefit, such as, "Physical therapy will improve your balance (or reduce the need for a cane)."

In a crisis, of course, you must do what you have to do, regardless of what he wants and no matter how grouchy he gets. If he can barely breathe but won't go to the emergency room, don't argue. Call an ambulance. If you feel intimidated by his protests, get over it. If it's a false alarm, so what? This is too important. You could be saving his life.

One client of mine, Lisa, wound up confiscating her husband's credit cards in order to keep him safe. It began when Billy, fifty-eight, took denial to new heights. During lengthy chemotherapy treatment, he persuaded Lisa to take a break and visit her family for a few days. He would stay with the aides she had hired. Exhausted, Lisa agreed.

After Lisa's departure, Billy, who was extremely ill and under quarantine to prevent infection, promptly sent the aides home. Although he was sixty pounds overweight and chemo had left him with little appetite, he loved food and had spent some time in his youth in New York City. He promptly picked up the phone and ordered a dozen overstuffed sandwiches and a large cheesecake flown in from the renowned Carnegie Delicatessen on Seventh Avenue. Then he called friend after friend to join him. Aware of his delicate condition, they declined.

Billy was a man who simply refused to be sick. He was determined to live his way, and no one was going to tell him differently, regardless of the toll on himself or on Lisa. Furious about the way he had endangered himself, Lisa took the only action she could and hid his credit card case.

8. Get him help for depression, if necessary.

Who doesn't feel "down" at times? A blue mood on occasion is a natural part of life. Depression, on the other hand, is different. It's serious, can complicate your partner's illness, inhibits the immune system, and increases his risk for suicide, heart disease, and other life-threatening problems. Yet male depression often goes undiagnosed or treated.

If you suspect he's depressed, and he is unable to accept his condition and mobilize his resources, try to seek medical help for him. Turn to a family doctor, psychiatrist, psychologist, clinical social worker, or other mental health professional. Medication, psychotherapy, or both may be indicated.

It may be an uphill battle to convince your mate to see a professional or take an antidepressant. Generally, men are more resistant to the idea of mental health treatment than women. The stigma of mental illness weighs heavily, and they worry that admitting they need help may affect their employment. Yet treatment with psychotherapy and/or medication is very effective for most depressed people. To encourage your partner to get help, cease nagging and realize that men don't like being labeled as depressed or noncompliant. In a calm, caring tone, try saying, "I'm concerned that you seem down," rather than, "Why are you so down all the time?" Remember, you don't want to sound like you're giving him orders. You can also appeal to his love for you. Tell him you need his help. If he won't go alone, perhaps he'll try couples therapy.

9. Suggest a support group.

Whether or not your partner is depressed, he may find a support group extremely helpful. If he can begin to talk about his worries and fears, he'll feel better, and it may relieve some of the tensions at home.

In one case, a husband in denial about his Parkinson's disease wouldn't consider a support group. He didn't want to be with sick people or see progression of the disease. Angry with him for his refusal, his wife decided to go to a support group herself. As she brought back information and talked about what she learned, she began to spark his interest. Eventually, he followed her lead and joined a Parkinson's disease patients group to learn from their experiences.

There are many reasons why a man may be reluctant to join a group. You can reach out to him and say something like, "I'm not sure how to help you. Have you thought about a support group?" Try adding, "Join a group for yourself, but it might help both of us cope with what's ahead." In the end, however, recognize that he has the right to decide for himself.

HELPING YOURSELF COPE WITH YOUR SICK PARTNER

SOMETIMES YOU DON'T know what your mate feels or needs. Men aren't taught to express their feelings, and most need help to do so. They may be more willing to talk about concrete physical problems, such as fatigue or sleep disturbances, than emotions like sadness, guilt, and fear. Yet most women have a positive impact on their men. We do get them to take better care of themselves than they would on their own, and sometimes we succeed in persuading them to stop harmful behavior. It's no accident that married men live longer than single males.

At the same time, your mate may behave in ways that try your patience. To cope, remember that he needs all the love and encouragement you can muster. It also helps to be flexible and to change as you need to—and consider a caregiver support group for yourself.

Reflections

- *Encourage your partner to focus on what he can do rather than on his limitations, and support his autonomy.*

- *Be good to yourself for his sake as well as yours. When you're exhausted, you're less able to deal with irritations.*

- *Help him talk about his feelings. Men don't like to discuss their illnesses, because they've been taught that doing so is a sign of weakness.*

- *Read between the lines and be alert to feelings of vulnerability that cause your mate to act mean or angry instead of appreciative.*

- *Denial is the most common male response to a health problem. Expect it and work around it.*

7

Educating Yourself about His Disease

If you've picked up this book, it probably isn't because you expect it to be a fun read. You're likely to be in a tough spot and looking for help. Coping with a mate's illness is a little like being Alice in Wonderland and falling down the rabbit hole. Suddenly what's up is down. Nothing is the same as it was before he became ill. Part of my goal is to help you settle yourself down enough to function—and that requires a foundation of solid information. In order to make the best decisions, you're going to have to learn all you can about your partner's condition.

Years ago, people put themselves in the doctor's hands and essentially said, "You're the boss. Tell me what to do." Today that doesn't work, because you're often expected to participate in medical decisions. Most physicians and other medical personnel perform best when you are an educated ally. They want your perspective, because you know the patient's habits, concerns, goals, and other details that count. And you are the one who will live with the results.

The world of medicine is also changing so rapidly that doctors can't know everything. You have a role to play in filling in the gaps. In chapter 2, for example, I told of a wife who tracked down a cure for her mate's agonizing skin condition that had appeared after cancer treatment. When nothing helped, including an expensive cream prescribed by the physician, this woman finally turned to the Internet. Online, she located a seven-dollar tube of cream that relieved her husband's suffering. Two months later, the condition had completely disappeared. The doctor, who had never heard of the cream, now recommends it to other patients.

You may not discover a miracle cure yourself, but you certainly can help your mate by becoming an inquiring, informed consumer as well as a powerful advocate for him. To play that role, you may have to overcome initial shyness or the wish for someone else to have all the answers.

You never planned to become an authority on your partner's illness. Piled on top of all the other things you have to do, you may feel overwhelmed at the thought of a cram course in heart disease or other diagnoses. If his condition has changed, you may need more information about complications—an advanced degree of sorts—at a time when you're worn out. But the more you know, the more control you have over what's going on, and the easier it is to map out effective strategies.

THE TIME FACTOR

A COMMON BARRIER to gathering information is the assumption that there is no time to do so. For example, my client Jodi panicked and started to cry when she was first told about her partner's diagnosis of leukemia. "I don't know what to do first," she exclaimed. In fact, nothing had to be done instantly. She had some time to educate herself and to see if her partner would consider getting a second opinion.

Take a deep breath and consider the situation. In most circumstances you have time to think, even though you may feel terrified. It is a crisis only in the case of an immediate life-threatening emergency, such as a heart attack or stroke. You know it's an immediate emergency if the onset is sudden and minutes or hours can make the difference between life and death or prevent severe impairment. Your partner needs medical attention *now*. Everything is fast-forwarded.

People often confuse true emergencies or crises with less immediate, but worrisome events. If your mate finds a testicular lump, or his routine annual checkup concludes with a nightmare diagnosis, that's a bad hit, a curve ball. Of course you're going to feel frightened, but you almost always have some time to think, plan, and educate yourself.

IS IT A TRUE EMERGENCY?

THE FOLLOWING signs warrant a trip to the emergency room or possibly a 911 call:

- Sudden chest pain or pain or pressure in upper abdomen
- Difficulty breathing, shortness of breath
- Sudden dizziness, faintness, weakness, vision change
- Severe or persistent vomiting or diarrhea
- Uncontrolled bleeding
- Difficulty speaking
- Suicidal feelings
- Confusion or changes in mental status
- Any sudden severe pain

Source: American College of Emergency Physicians

The task is to slow down rather than allow fear to distort your judgment. Unanswered questions may be difficult to tolerate, and anxiety can push you into hasty decisions on the spot. Instead, take the time you need to examine options and act thoughtfully. You want to conserve your energy, and in the long run some careful planning may save you unnecessary steps. When you realize you can buy time to evaluate choices and get input from others, you relieve some of the pressure on yourself.

Slow Onset Illness

Not every illness suddenly explodes into your life, changing everything. Some conditions unfold slowly and gradually. For example, very small, subtle symptoms can signal the beginning of a neurological condition. It may take time to fully digest the implications and admit that something is wrong. Awareness of Parkinson's disease or multiple sclerosis may start with a mistyped word, a finger that won't move when it should, or a series of surprise falls.

This actually happened to one of my clients. He noticed that his pinky wouldn't type the letter he wanted—and instantly knew something was wrong. In another case, an athletic client began to trip when climbing stairs. The cause turned out to be a tumor in his spine.

Diagnosis may be elusive and time-consuming, with tests and more tests to rule out other conditions, and misdiagnoses do happen. This is a stressful, anxiety-producing process, because you can't start learning about the disease and working toward treatment or a cure until the illness has a name and you know what you're dealing with.

One wife, Nancy, was concerned about her husband's increasing balance problems. Certain that the reason was excessive alcohol consumption, she started to nag him to quit drinking. I finally convinced the couple to see a doctor. The diagnosis:

Parkinson's disease. This is a typical bad news/good news situation. The bad news was that he had a slow but progressive disease. The good news was that now that he knew what he was facing, he willingly reduced his drinking. She stopped nagging and went into high gear to find ways to help him live longer with a better quality of life.

The upside of a slow-onset illness is that you have plenty of time to find information about the course of the disease, absorb it, and make measured decisions. You have some idea of what to expect and perhaps can prepare for what may lie ahead. For example, in multiple sclerosis, there may be attacks and remissions. Acute episodes can involve double vision, numbness in limbs, or other symptoms. Advance knowledge reduces uncertainty and helps calm you down.

AFTER THE DIAGNOSIS

THE INTERNET AND other resources are available to help you make educated decisions. Take advantage of them.

Talk with Your Doctor

You may be sitting in the doctor's office or a hospital room when you hear the news. Your heart may pound, and you may feel stunned or even panicked. Or perhaps you react with paralysis. Hopefully, you'll find a way to break through the fear, despite what you feel inside, and get answers to basic questions, such as, "What is the stage of the disease?" "What's the prognosis?" "What are the treatment options?"

If the doctor knows your husband's case well, he or she is your primary source of information. Today, however, you have access to additional medical information on an unprecedented scale. The physician's explanation can be supplemented with research online and elsewhere.

Consult the Internet

As many as 52 million American adults have turned to the Internet for health or medical information, according to the Pew Internet & American Life Project. And 54 percent of them search to help a family member or friend—often to obtain additional data following a doctor's visit. Online research can also help you figure out the questions you want to ask the doctor before the next visit.

Women are the biggest users of online health and medical research, and of course the convenience is unbeatable. The computer is a shortcut to instant answers. You can sit down anytime—even at three a.m. if you can't sleep—and find what you need.

For starters, on sites like www.healthfinder.gov and www.nlm .nih.gov, you can ground yourself in the basics of an illness and its treatment options. Other sites provide information about the best doctors and hospitals to handle his condition. Of course, in a 911 emergency, the hospital decision may be out of your hands. Your partner probably goes to the nearest facility, although it never hurts to ask if there is a more suitable alternative. But in other cases, there are choices.

When Florence's husband suffered a stroke years ago, they were at their weekend place in upstate New York. The ambulance took him to a small local hospital. Florence called her family physician in Manhattan to discuss whether (and when) transfer to a major teaching hospital was advisable. "I wanted to maximize my husband's chances for a good recovery," she recalls. The doctor agreed with her thinking and proceeded to research the best facility for stroke in New York City. Later he called back to recommend transfer as soon as her husband's condition stabilized. Today, there are many primary stroke centers in the United States. You can locate the closest one at www.StrokeAssociation.org.

The Internet is also a good place to find out what to expect during and after treatment, including side effects. When you're managing a chronic condition, you can glean information on exercise and nutrition, medications available as cheaper generics, and gadgets and equipment that can improve your partner's quality of life at home. Support groups can be found online. You can also connect with others in similar situations through chat rooms and e-mail discussion groups.

Beware of the Downside

Unfortunately, the Internet has its drawbacks. It can drown you in facts, making it impossible to absorb it all. When presented with so many choices, you may want to throw up your hands. The Internet can also force-feed information you're not ready for and don't want. If your mate's condition is in its early stages, it's often scary to read about advanced cases.

For these reasons, and because there's a lot of misinformation online, make sure you are using a reputable, authoritative site. (See page 113 for what to look for.) It's also wise to get your physician's perspective. While researching her husband's case, one wife saw pictures online of a frightening complication. Worry that the same complication could happen to him kept her up at night for weeks until she finally confided her fear to the doctor. He assured her the complication was extremely rare, putting her mind at ease.

Other people may try to be their own doctors. In her book *Surviving Healthcare,* Pamela Armstrong, MPH, MBA, a health care industry insider, warns: "Some consumers use information from the Internet and other sources to self-diagnose and determine the treatment they need. They then try to find a physician who will give them what they have decided they need." This does nobody any good and undermines the team effort you're trying to achieve with the doctor. As is true of many research tools, the Internet must be handled with care.

CLINICAL TRIALS

PATIENT STUDIES are conducted today for many diseases to evaluate new treatments, ways to improve patients' quality of life, methods of prevention, and for other purposes. You can ask your doctor about trials that might benefit your mate, or find them on the Internet through Web sites for the National Institutes of Health (NIH) or disease-specific organizations, such as the American Cancer Society.

It can be difficult to decide whether the best option is a clinical trial or standard treatment. The upside of a clinical trial is that your partner may receive otherwise unavailable medication. The downside is that he may get a placebo. It's always a gamble. To help weigh the pros and cons and find out if your mate is eligible for a particular trial, talk to your physician and other medical authorities. You may want to get a second opinion or consult family members for their input as well.

When You Need Computer Help

Despite the pervasiveness of online resources, not everyone feels comfortable (or competent) using them. If you're technologically challenged and feel intimidated, or don't have access to a computer, this is the time to ask someone who is computer-savvy to research online for you. A volunteer fell in the lap of one lucky Denver wife, Helene. She felt shell-shocked when her husband's non-Hodgkin's lymphoma recurred and he required a bone marrow transplant. She had recently reconnected with an old neighbor after a chance meeting at the supermarket. The neighbor, who had just helped her father through prostate cancer treatment, told her, "I know how to do medical research and who to contact. I just did it. Let me handle this for you."

Helene recalls, "She did all this research for me at a time when I just couldn't. I had two preschoolers *and* a husband with a huge slice in his groin who really couldn't get around. I got a copy of the pathology report, gave it to her, and she took it from there. What a wonderful gift!"

If you're not as fortunate, think about people you know who are proficient online—the student next door, your nephew, stepdaughter, or grandchild. Or tell your church or other place of worship what you need. Chances are, members can help. Libraries remain another resource. They have computers, and staff who can help you with online research.

Other Sources of Information

As helpful as Internet research can be, it is not the only way to learn what you need to know. Look for articles and books on your man's disease at the library. The pharmacist can provide information on drug interactions and other issues. Virtually every illness has a knowledgeable support organization, such as the American Heart Association, American Diabetes Association, American Cancer Society, American Stroke Association, and National Kidney Foundation. Such organizations offer a wealth of information on the disease, the latest advances, and services to patients and families. You can connect with them online or reach local chapters by phone. (See the Resources section at the end of this book for contact information.)

SECOND OPINIONS:
PART OF YOUR RESEARCH

WHEN YOUR PARTNER is ill, there's almost always more than one expert and treatment option available. Although getting a second opinion can seem like a needless, time-consuming extra step, and it sometimes confuses you, it is usually worth the challenge. (It may also be required by your health insurance.) One client of mine regrets not seeking a second opinion after her husband's diagnosis of early-stage colorectal cancer. Surgery alone was recommended. Although radiation to shrink the tumor first was mentioned, it was ruled out as unnecessary. "That was exactly what we wanted to hear. We felt so devastated by the diagnosis at the time that we couldn't have coped with the idea of radiation *plus* surgery," the wife recalled.

In fact, the tumor turned out to be larger and more advanced than expected, and the surgery left the husband with severe chronic issues. "He probably wouldn't have had those problems if he had had radiation first. We'll never know for sure, but we'll always wonder whether another doctor would have recommended it—and saved my husband a lifetime of trouble," she says.

In my experience, this reluctance to look further is common. The very process of getting a second opinion creates anxiety. First it takes time to find another specialist and get an appointment. You live in a gray zone of uncertainty for weeks or even months. You may be afraid that your doctor will be mad at you for checking elsewhere. Some people also feel uncomfortable making their own decisions. What do you do if the second opinion disagrees with the first?

This is when it's most important to act like an adult. You may want to collapse and be taken care of—and you have every reason to feel like running away. But if you do that, who will be the wise one? If you feel too overwhelmed to focus, get someone to help you make the calls or ask the questions. Most people are reassured by getting a second opinion.

LEARN WITH YOUR MATE IF YOU CAN

OFTEN YOU AND your partner are able to work and learn together. When this is possible, it lightens your load and is also a way to bond and share. Each of you may have different research strengths, such as advanced computer skills or the ability to ask the right questions. Together you may make a strong team.

I remember a Baltimore woman, Abby, who was desperate to improve her husband's quality of life. Online, she found a doctor in Oklahoma noted for research in his condition. She handed her husband the contact information. He took it from there and proceeded to call the doctor and leave a message. To Abby's surprise, the doctor called back in a few hours, intrigued by the case. Previous test results and other information were faxed back and forth. Eventually they agreed on an in-person appointment. "My husband had the 'can-do' attitude of a businessman, and he got fast results. I would have put off calling and obsessed that the doctor would never call a stranger back," said Abby.

The couple flew to Oklahoma to see the physician and found the visit well worth the trip. Abby recalled, "He spent two hours with us, talking, testing, and explaining. There was no quick fix, but he had a fresh perspective, and there were options we hadn't heard about before. We came back renewed. How do you place a price on hope?"

Your mate can be a particular help in a long-term illness that involves a lot of complicated information. You're inundated with so many medical terms you don't understand, and there are multiple options and opinions. How do you sort out the best ones?

One young couple educated themselves methodically when tests revealed the husband had a specific cancer gene and was therefore at high risk for additional malignancies. The couple faced a number of very difficult decisions. The wife, a very organized woman, was able to use her talent for list making to help her husband. She categorized and even color coded her own reference book detailing the doctors and other medical professionals she spoke with, the topic talked about, and highlights of the discussion. Making lists and gathering information helped her handle her own anxiety—and become a useful advocate for him.

LEARNING WHILE UNDER FIRE: SIX STEPS TO GOOD DECISION MAKING

TO MAKE GOOD decisions, you need reliable facts. The challenge is to gather the information even when you may feel afraid and overburdened. Here's how to proceed:

1. **Ask your doctor to explain and interpret.**

   Your husband's physician can help you sort out what is helpful information from what is not. He or she can translate data, such as survival statistics, and put the information into the proper context. The odds may frighten and depress you, but they are only numbers. They may not apply to your mate. You can save yourself a lot of anguish by getting the facts for his individual case.

   Research needs interpretation, too. A new study may get lots of press attention, but there may be questions about who can be helped, what the results really mean, and whether they are flawed as a result of the way the research was conducted. The trick is to learn what you can, yet keep an open mind and resist swallowing the implications whole.

   Remember to check with the doctor, too, before your mate tries a complementary or alternative medication (CAM). Eastern and Western medicines are meeting in today's world. It's common to turn to the Internet for instant information on herbal products, vitamins, and minerals—or to read about them in other media, or hear about them through word-of-mouth. A friend raves about a remedy she bought at the health food store. But such products can have dangerous, even life-threatening, interactions with prescribed drugs, including some heart medications. Many complementary or alternative medications help people, but medical care can be complicated. Ask questions first.

2. Check reliability of online sites.

Eighty-six percent of people who get medical information through the Internet worry about how reliable it is, and with good reason. Ask these questions when you visit an online site:

- *Who sponsors it?* Is it a medical center, like the Mayo Clinic; a renowned facility for the disease, like Joslin Diabetes Center/Joslin Clinic; a medical school; a government agency, like the National Institutes of Health (NIH) or the Centers for Disease Control (CDC)? Is it a respected organization, like the American Heart Association?

- *What's the source of the information?* Is it research-based, or simply advice from someone? For example, NIH now has a National Center for Complementary and Alternative Medicine (NCCAM). Its Web site (www.nccam.nih.gov) is an excellent place for authoritative information on therapies. Consult the National Cancer Institute's Office of Cancer Complementary and Alternative Medicine (OCCAM) site (www.cancer .gov/cam). Try www.arthritis.org, the Arthritis Foundation's Web site, for tips on alternative treatments that might help arthritis patients, such as dietary supplements that relieve pain.

- *How current is the information?* Is it regularly updated?

■ *Can you contact the site sponsor to ask questions?* It's helpful if you find you need more information.

■ *What information about you is required?* Do you have to become a member to access information, and what happens to the personal information you supply if you do join?

3. **Become familiar with the vocabulary.**

When you read or hear medical terminology you don't understand, don't let it pass. Ask, "What's that?" or look it up online or in a medical dictionary. Each disease has some of its own jargon. It helps to learn enough of the terminology to communicate effectively with medical professionals and fully understand what they are talking about. Think of it as visiting a foreign country. In order to find your way around and avoid getting lost, you have to learn certain language basics. If this is not your gift, find someone who can help you.

For example, did you know *dialysis* is the process of cleaning wastes from the body artificially? *Chronic obstructive pulmonary disease* (COPD) refers to chronic bronchitis and emphysema. An *oncologist* is a cancer specialist. A *blood count* is a measurement of the number of red cells, white cells, and platelets in a blood sample. Keep a list of necessary terms so that you can refer back to it.

4. **Keep up your education.**

Learning about a chronic illness is never really over. Lawyers, psychologists, and others take courses to stay current and retain their certification. It's wise for you to keep up with the latest news and advances in your mate's illness as well. Sometimes the outlook for his condition can change surprisingly fast. I recall one client who was told that if his cancer recurred, nothing could be done. Five years later he had a recurrence scare, and he and his wife assumed he was going to die. But the scare turned out to be just that; there was no cancer. Later on, in the course of discussing the false alarm with a surgeon, they mentioned their escape from a death sentence. The surgeon was shocked. "Oh no," he hastened to explain. "There's a whole lot we can do for a recurrence today." The couple had no idea that effective new treatments had become available.

After an emergency, if your mate is at high risk for another attack, learn all you can about the symptoms to watch for. For example, stroke is the leading cause of long-term disability in the United States, and stroke patients are at high risk for subsequent strokes. Emergency room treatment within three hours can significantly reduce or prevent impairment. Take the time now to educate yourself for possible future incidents. For example, signs of stroke include sudden numbness or weakness of the face, arm, or leg; sudden difficulty speaking, or confusion; sudden vision loss in one or both eyes; and sudden severe headache for unknown reasons.

Doctors may forget to tell you that about 20 percent of heart disease patients suffer from major depression, which can boost the risk of another heart attack. If you're alert to this fact, you can watch for symptoms of your partner's depression. (See pages 85–87 and 96–97 for further information on male depression.) If depression occurs, treatment reduces his risk for another coronary and helps both of you survive what might otherwise be an extremely difficult time.

Learn about ways to improve your mate's quality of life. If he has a chronic condition like diabetes or an ostomy, educate yourself to all the equipment necessary and take advantage of catalog or manufacturer hotlines that can answer questions and provide tips.

5. Use backup help.

A relative or friend who is an MD, nurse, or other medical practitioner—or someone who has experienced the same condition firsthand—can help you put information in perspective. Take advantage of the person's expertise. It's additional informal, reliable information that can bring you peace of mind. Florence's cousin, an internist, has played that role for her often. Although he lives several states away, he's been a sounding board and a lifeline at times when she's felt confused and afraid. "It's such a relief to be able to call and say, 'What's your take?'" she says.

6. Be kind to yourself.

How you get through this medical crash course depends in large part on you and your attitude. Some people are open to learning as much as possible. They are curious and want full information. If you are not this type of person, try looking at learning in a new way— as a route to power. Although your particular experience is unique, use the knowledge that is already available. Realize that there is no such thing as perfection. You're not going to get an "A." All you can do is your best, but your best may be much better than you thought.

The one thing you *can't* do is nothing. If you feel too confused or anxious to focus on fact-finding when you are in the midst of dealing with an illness, and are having trouble educating yourself, recognize that you probably can do it well enough with help. Perhaps a friend or family member can act as a coach and guide and motivate you when you lose confidence. If that doesn't work, then someone has to do it for you. Part of being effective is knowing when to turn to others.

Reflections

- *Try to learn as much as you can about your mate's illness.*

- *Unless it's a true crisis or emergency, you can usually buy time to gather information and think things through.*

- *Take advantage of the Internet and other resources.*

- *Beware of misinformation online and misinterpreting data.*

- *Remember, knowledge is strength and control.*

8

Dealing with the Medical Establishment

It's eight a. m. at the doctor's office. "How are you feeling?" the physician asks your husband. The answer is a grunted "Okay," when in fact he had a gigantic anxiety attack at breakfast (a repeat of the one yesterday), and he feels so shaky he wants to stay home from the office today. So *you* speak up and explain what's really going on.

The doctor immediately responds. "It's the—," he says, indicating the new medication he prescribed last week. He proceeds to reduce the dosage. Within a day or two, your husband's anxiety is gone.

It seems hard to believe that someone wouldn't mention a debilitating new symptom to the doctor, but just stop for a minute and think. Your mate may be trying to cope with a chronic condition that chips away at his quality of life, with a threatening diagnosis, or with impending surgery. No matter how much bravado he displays, remember, deep down he is probably scared to death and not thinking clearly—especially if he feels out of control. This is where male denial so often surfaces. If he doesn't say out loud that he feels terrible, in his mind the anxiety isn't really happening.

Additionally, your partner is frequently in no condition to protect his best interests, which is why he needs an advocate and liaison between him and the medical staff and system. Whether you welcome that role or not, that person is you. In the doctor's office, the hospital, taking outpatient tests, or in treatment, it has now become your responsibility to help your mate get what he needs.

YOUR ROLE AT THE DOCTOR'S OFFICE

AS UPSET AS you may be, you are not the patient. Therefore it is up to you to be the best fact finder, comforter, advocate, and secretary you can. Remember your coping style and lean into your strengths. (See chapter 3.)

Don't Let Your Partner Go Alone

Robyn faced a situation like the one described at the beginning of this chapter. She had almost skipped the doctor's appointment and let her husband go alone, because she wanted to attend an early meeting at work. "It's a good thing I changed my mind," she muses. "Joshua might still be having anxiety attacks if I hadn't."

Try to make sure that someone accompanies your partner to important medical visits. Whether or not he admits it, he's probably nervous like everyone else in his situation. When he talks to the doctor, he might be stressed and forget to ask important questions. If he remembers to ask, he may not completely recall the answers and be able to relay them to you later. He may think he doesn't need an advocate along at these times, but the truth is, he does. Your presence helps him feel supported by someone who loves him and is in his corner.

If you truly cannot go with him, ask someone else to substitute. I know firsthand how important this can be, because I once had my own cancer scare. My husband couldn't go with me to see the doctor, and my eldest daughter took his place. Later, when my husband asked, "What did the doctor say?" I couldn't respond coherently. (Yes, even professionals need help.) Fortunately, my daughter did remember, and the physician was considerate enough to repeat everything when my husband called to get clarification.

There are cases where the first and best choice is a surrogate, such as another family member. Some partners are so anxious that their presence compounds stress, and it's better that they stay home. At such times a man might want to take a close buddy with him. Men rarely reach out to others, and the appointment gives them a chance to bond in new ways.

Making the Most of Appointment Time

Because you see things differently than your mate does, you may be better at communicating with the doctor. Yet you may be nervous, too. Rather than rely on your memory, try to arrive at the appointment with a list of questions and topics you want to discuss, ranked in order of importance. Then your key concerns will be addressed even if there isn't enough time to talk about everything on your mind. You'll save confusion later if you keep pad and pen in hand (or even bring a personal organizer or laptop) to record all the relevant information and instructions from the doctor.

When the appointment involves a new diagnosis or treatment, it helps to ask in advance whether the doctor will provide printed information to read before you talk together. If so, you can arrive early to look through the brochures as you sit in the waiting room. When faced with potentially disturbing news, your mate may be too tense to read and absorb the information. He may get up and pace or zone out. You may even want to join him.

The Art of Asking Questions

Despite all the advice we've heard about taking responsibility and being assertive, many people remain awed and intimidated by medical doctors as authority figures. Such reactions interfere with getting information and help. What's often forgotten is the fact that you pay physicians to perform a service for you. Your mate may be the one in need, but the doctor works for him (and for you as his advocate), not the other way around. Ultimately, you and your partner are in charge.

Says Robyn, "My husband would ask questions at work if he didn't understand something about a project, but it's different when his body is the issue—even though he wants to know. The doctor is this godlike expert, and whatever he or she says must be right. So I have to ask, 'Can we try this?' or, 'What about that?' I also learned not to give up if the answer is no. You're entitled to say, 'Tell me why.'"

When explanations are not a physician's strength, you may have to prod or ask a nurse or another, more communicative member of the medical team. One wife realized her husband's surgeon was great at operating but not at talking. She turned to their family physician, who was happy to answer questions and fill in gaps.

Be prepared for the possibility that your husband may not appreciate your persistence and may become annoyed with you. He may feel embarrassed, especially if the doctor glances at him with an unspoken "What's wrong with her?" If that happens, bear up. This does *not* mean you should stop asking questions. You're likely to be thanked for your efforts later on.

Developing Personal Rapport

You do want your mate to be more than just a number, so be cordial with the physicians. If the doctor is male, your mate may be able to establish a personal bond by talking sports or the stock market. If he isn't the type to engage in such conversation, maybe you can find a way to break the ice yourself. The photos on the wall in the office may trigger a comment such as, "I see you have a lovely family." Then the doctor mentions an upcoming trip to Disney World, and a light conversation is up and running. Each time you have an appointment, ask briefly about the children (or the dog). This sets you apart from everyone else in the waiting room and can give you an edge. For example, the physician may give you a private cell phone number or tell the receptionist it's okay to be interrupted when you call.

HOW TO TALK TO THE DOCTOR

- *Bring relevant information.* If this is a first appointment, remember that the visit works two ways. The physician needs input from you. Bring along your mate's medical history and a list of his medications and dosages, including both prescription and nonprescription medicines, supplements, and vitamins.

- *Keep asking until the answers are clear.* If you don't understand the explanations, rephrase them—for example, "Doctor, do you mean—?" Then you can follow up with, "Can you explain further?" or "What exactly do you mean?" And don't forget, "What if—?" Collaborate with your mate on which questions are most important, too.

- *Do your homework.* Learn about your mate's condition and the medical jargon connected with it so that you can talk knowledgeably.

> • *Be diplomatic.* If you want your partner to try a new
> medication or an alternative treatment you've heard
> about, tell the physician something like, "I wonder
> what you think about—." The doctor is the expert and
> should be treated as one. However, if an idea you think
> has merit is vetoed, consider a second opinion.

Dealing with Other Personnel

Make questions a habit, too, when talking with office staff and other personnel. In one case, a man successfully treated for cancer had a follow-up CAT scan. His wife recounts, "We got a call afterward from the radiologist's office saying they needed his old CAT scans—and my heart stopped. I was terrified that meant he had a recurrence. I finally called the oncologist and said, 'You need to find out what's going on.' It turned out it was nothing. They said, 'Oh, everything was fine. We just wanted to compare the scans.' It would have saved me so much anguish if I had only asked, 'Why do you want the old CAT scans?'"

At other times the challenge is to ask for what you need. In her book *Love, Honor, & Value,* Suzanne Geffen Mintz, president of the National Family Caregivers Association, speaks of inconsiderate treatment at the doctor's office. Personnel would leave her and her husband, who has multiple sclerosis, on their own to hoist him from his wheelchair to the examining table. A small woman, Mintz couldn't help much. She learned to call in advance of an appointment and state, "My husband is in a wheelchair. Are there people available who can help him transfer? We'll need some strong arms to help us." She advises, "One of the criteria for choosing health professionals should be the way they deal with disabilities. When my husband and I went to a chiropractor, we discovered his office wasn't wheelchair accessible. We never went back."

You want to see someone who makes life easy for you. When visiting a practitioner for the first time, it's wise to call in advance to check on accessibility for the disabled. At other times the issue may be receptionists who are always too busy talking with one another to tend to you or who mix up your tests or appointments.

When staff is repeatedly incompetent or rude, it's important to let the physician know. Explain in terms of "I feel ignored here" or "I don't feel respected." If nothing changes, you can always go elsewhere.

SUPPORTING YOUR PARTNER IN THE HOSPITAL

HOSPITALS ARE PLACES where your mate is a temporary visitor—at a time when he's scared, confused, stripped of his dignity, often in pain, or possibly even unconscious. Both of you are strangers in a strange land. In this intimidating environment, he needs you more than ever as his champion. Although hospitals ask about insurance first, your job is to focus on care first and enlist everyone's cooperation. You're on a learning curve, because hospitals have a culture all their own.

The Cast of Characters

The first step in getting the best possible care and related services is to know what everybody's duties are and how they can help you.

Your mate's doctor: The attending physician is the one who admits him, coordinates care, and is well informed about what goes on at the hospital. He or she is the one to talk with if you feel things aren't going right.

Nurses: Establish a cordial relationship with the nurses who are responsible for day-to-day care. That may be more difficult than it sounds, because nurses may be temporaries or work only three days in a row (on longer shifts). Just as you're getting to know the person, you may have to start all over again with someone else. Although this is frustrating, it is worth the effort to be friendly.

A nurse's kindness and willingness to go the extra mile for your partner is priceless, whether it's moving just a little faster to bring the pain medication or taking a few minutes to sit and hold his hand when he's feeling afraid and you're not there. Nurses can also be valuable resources for another reason. A long time ago, someone told me, "If you want to find a good doctor, ask a nurse to recommend one. Nurses know."

Case manager: This person follows the patient from admission to discharge, making sure your mate's needs are met. If you're wondering about his status and weren't present at doctors' rounds, the case manager is an excellent person to ask, "Help me understand what's going on?" The case manager also stays in touch with the insurance company to work through any coverage problems.

Social worker: Make friends with the social worker, who understands what you're going through and is there to meet psychological, social, and other patient and family needs. This person can steer you to additional services, including financial assistance, and help you find out whether you're eligible for entitlements like Medicaid or Medicare. The social worker can also connect you with a caregiver group within the hospital or outside it. A case manager or social worker arranges for discharge, but you don't want to wait until the last minute. Talk with this person early to smooth out any potential problems in advance.

When I was taking care of a seriously ill family member, it was the hospital social worker's simple question, "Who's taking care of *you*?" that brought me to tears. It took an outside professional to remind me that I didn't have to do it all alone.

Patient representative: This person is there to serve as a liaison between you and the hospital and cut through red tape. The rep can also arrange for an interpreter, or for hotel accommodations if you are from out of town. One client remembers how a patient representative helped her through the agony of sitting in a waiting room while her mate was undergoing a coronary bypass. As Mary paced, her rep contacted her hourly to keep her posted on the progress of surgery. The person brought out a cart of tea, coffee, and sandwiches, which made a terrifying experience less stressful and more humane.

In another case, a wife had trouble getting copies of her husband's X-rays. During this time, she received a call from the patient rep about a billing issue and grabbed the opportunity to get help. She said, "I'm sure medical records will pay more attention to you than me. Could you call and see what you can do about the X-rays?" The person called back in minutes to say, "Come and get 'em."

Your Partner Needs Your Protection

Many kinds of help surround you in the hospital, but so does the potential for trouble. Although I deal with the medical establishment all the time in my work and have a healthy respect for hospitals, I know that even though they are beneficial, they can sometimes be dangerous places when you're ill.

I don't wish to frighten you, but look at the statistics. Drug errors, such as incorrect dosages or administering the wrong medications, impair or kill almost eight hundred thousand people a year in U.S. hospitals. One of your jobs is to know the drugs your mate is taking and check that he's getting what he should. You can't just assume that this is true, because mistakes happen more often than we might think. For example, one night a patient asked for something to help him sleep. When his wife arrived the next morning, she found him in a state of confusion and agitation. She complained to the doctor, who proceeded to prescribe a different pill. Yet the following day, her husband had grown even more disoriented, not less. "It was very scary. He was mumbling and stumbling," she recalls. "They had given him the same sleep medication once again instead of the replacement. The change order was never executed."

During the same hospital stay, another necessary medication was skipped two different times for an entire day because of glitches. It took this wife's badgering to reinstate it. "They probably thought I was a pain, but so what? My husband's well-being was at stake," she said.

In addition, infections contracted while in the hospital affect even more people—roughly two million patients a year. About ninety thousand patients die of them, according to the Centers for Disease Control (CDC). At the very least, try to notice whether personnel (doctors included) have washed or used a disinfectant on their hands before tending to your mate or performing a procedure. If in doubt, feel free to ask. Wash your own hands, too.

When I was in the hospital for surgery, my daughters, who had just read an article on preventing hospital-acquired infections, cleaned my room and the equipment in it with an antiseptic solution. Later I told my surgeon about it, who not only thought it was an excellent idea, but also asked me to write to the hospital board to help lobby for more funds for the cleaning staff.

Demystifying the Technology

Hospitals are a mysterious environment. Your mate is surrounded by strange equipment, buzzing sounds, bleeps, and blinking lights. It's important to learn what you can about all the gear and gadgets. Catheters, IVs, ventilating masks, and other technology can make his room look like an IBM computer command center. That doesn't mean you have to remain in the dark. As you sit in his room all those hours, ask nurses and other personnel walking in and out to explain what each tube, beep, and needle accomplishes or signifies. Then you won't panic every time you hear a strange sound, but you *will* know when a nurse is needed pronto. You can also get preliminary education in how to operate equipment your mate may need later at home.

YOUR EMOTIONAL FUEL TANK

YOU HAVE TO spend time in the hospital to support your mate, but you owe it to both of you to admit the limits of your emotional energy—and ration accordingly. My limits are different from yours, because we all have different personalities and different kinds of marriages or committed relationships. Some couples are bonded at the hip, doing everything together; others are very independent, with separate interests and friends; some fall in between.

If time together is primary, you may do well sitting at his bedside day and night. Just his presence is enough. But if you have children to care for or lead a relatively independent life, the experience of togetherness 24/7 may stifle you.

Honor and accept your relationship without feeling guilty. Heather confessed that when she got home from the hospital at night, she felt so exhausted she turned her cell phone off to prevent her husband from calling to complain about the night nurses. "I couldn't stand it anymore. I had to unwind and get a good night's sleep so I could get up and go back there the next morning. I felt, 'He's in the hospital. Let them take care of him until morning. I have nothing left to give.'" If your partner truly needs someone there more often, call upon family and friends to fill in for you.

Respecting your limits can actually be a lifesaver. As I mentioned in chapter 1, research shows that your risk of death increases when your mate is hospitalized for serious illness, especially during the first thirty days, when stress is high and so many initial adjustments in your life must be made. This fact underlines how important it is to take care of yourself.

GETTING WHAT YOU NEED AT DISCHARGE

WHEN YOUR PARTNER is ready to come home, it's a relief to know you won't have to yo-yo back and forth to the hospital anymore. It's also natural to worry about taking care of him all by yourself, without the nurses' station right down the hall. There's no way to escape all of your concerns. If you're human, you're going to have some. But you can ward off unwarranted panic by asking useful questions before discharge:

1. **What home care help will I get—and for how long?**
   Home care offers nursing, physical or speech therapy, and assistance with daily living activities like bathing, dressing, and shopping. The kinds of help you get—and how long you get it—varies depending on your insurance and the situation. The social worker or case manager arranging for discharge can tell you what coverage you've got. You can also ask around about the best home health agency to provide care. Even if the hospital recommends an agency, you don't have to accept the recommendation.

2. **How can I effectively manage his condition?**
   What tasks will you have to perform, such as wound care? How much instruction will you get?

3. **What signs of trouble should I watch for, and what should I do if they occur?**

   All sorts of "what if's" are likely to torment you. What if your partner's wound gets infected? What if he starts hemorrhaging? These are critical questions to get answers to in advance.

4. **Will any special medical or other equipment be required at home, and am I covered for it?**

   Will your mate need a wheelchair or walker, for example? You also want an emergency number to call in case the overnight feed pump starts beeping at three a.m.

5. **Is he being discharged to another facility?**

   Sometimes a patient goes first to a subacute or rehabilitation facility rather than directly home. If so, what's the best one in your area and what length of stay is anticipated? Visit a few in person and compare them when you have a choice.

What about Recovery Time?

One of the doctor's jobs is to help your mate remain positive, but beware of an overly optimistic estimate of recuperation time. It may take a lot longer than you're led to believe. For example, people often aren't prepared for the long recovery after a heart attack. Most doctors want to be encouraging and may tell your partner, "Oh, you'll be up and running in a few weeks," when it frequently takes much longer. If your husband isn't back on his feet fast, he doesn't understand why he's so ill. You may have to push to get a realistic assessment of what to expect. If necessary, ask others you know who have been through the experience, or check an online illness-related chat room for an accurate picture, keeping in mind that every case is different.

Realistically, recovery from major surgery may take weeks or months, depending on the circumstances. After all, your mate may experience psychological changes and may also mourn the loss of a body part or function. Depression often occurs after prostate cancer surgery. He may not feel well and may obsess over his lack of sexual desire, or even more directly, he may question whether his penis will ever work again. It's only natural for him to feel depressed, moody, or upset.

This is your time to be supportive of your mate and ask for the truth from the doctor. If you thought your partner would be back to his old self by now, it's important to ask, "Is this normal or not?" It's true that if physicians told you everything to expect, you might worry needlessly. If they don't tell, they leave you unprepared.

Is Your Partner Being Discharged Too Early?

The average hospital stay in the United States is only 4.8 days, according to the Centers for Disease Control (CDC), and we often hear about patients being pushed out of the hospital too quickly. In fact, there is an association between early discharge and poor mental health in caregivers. It's frightening and stressful if you have to assume responsibilities that ordinarily belong to a nurse when your medical expertise only runs to iodine and Band-Aids.

You may think your partner is too sick or weak to leave the hospital. If insurance won't cover a longer stay, there are appeal procedures you can follow. One wife flatly refused to take her husband home only twenty-four hours after he received a defibrillator. As a result, he was allowed to stay an extra day.

SIX WAYS TO GUARD YOUR PARTNER'S INTERESTS (AND YOURS)

THERE'S SO MUCH you can't control as you move through the medical system. Yet you often have more power than you think. Here's how to maximize help and services along the way:

1. **Choose a doctor who's a good fit.**

    Although the perfect doctor may be hard to find, you want a physician both you and your mate feel comfortable working with. He or she should be willing and able to step in on your behalf when a problem arises in or out of the hospital. The doctor's manner counts mightily. Expect respect and a good listener. The last thing you want is someone who talks down to your husband, lectures him like a child, or behaves like a steamroller. If your mate doesn't trust and feel compatible with his doctor, his recovery can be impaired.

    There are many jokes about surgeons' lack of friendly bedside manner, which regretfully are based on some reality. Surgeons are usually hired for their ability, not their charm. If the surgeon in your case is the best around but seems cold or arrogant, you may want to use him or her but find emotional support elsewhere. Perhaps the surgeon's nurse or other staff can be more understanding.

    If it's any consolation, when medical professionals become patients themselves, even they sometimes complain about the way they're treated. In one case, a hematologist had to retire because of his emphysema. His wife, a nurse herself, recalls, "It was generally an advantage to be medical professionals, although not always.

Doctors talk to you differently. They don't have to explain the basics, because you know everything. But when I asked one physician a question, he said, 'I can't believe you don't know that.' What a jerk he was!"

2. Work with your team.

It often takes several health professionals to get (or keep) your mate well or maximize his functioning. For example, the team for an arthritis patient might involve a primary care doctor, rheumatologist, orthopedic surgeon, physiatrist, podiatrist, or ophthalmologist. If he's had a colostomy, the team may include a colorectal surgeon, gastroenterologist, stoma nurse, nutritionist, and, if requested, even an acupuncturist. Regardless of the lineup for your mate, both of you want to work closely with these people for the best possible outcome. The National Family Caregivers Association offers local workshops on communicating effectively with health professionals. See the Resources section at the back of this book for contact information.

3. Act in advance.

If you know that your partner is going to the hospital and has time to prepare, check the details of your insurance coverage for the hospital stay, home care, rehabilitation, and so forth if they are necessary. Handling insurance claims is intimidating—there's all that fine print. But better to wade through them now than to wind up with unpleasant surprises about coverage later. If you are part of an HMO (health maintenance organization) that doesn't permit out-of-network choices of doctors and services, you may have to find your way to HMO executives who will tell you how to appeal, or heads of hospital departments who will tell you who's best for the task at hand or, if necessary, who will pull strings for you. Sometimes you may have to ask a case manager or social worker to intervene. Although your choices in your plan may be limited, you may have more options than you realize. In a PPO (preferred provider organization), by definition, you have more choices already built in.

Talk to the case manager or social worker before discharge to buy time to smooth out any problems that may arise.

4. Speak up.

It's up to you to protect your mate's interests at the doctor's office, in the hospital, and after discharge. You may have to do it without help from him, and a combination of assertiveness and diplomacy may be necessary. Such skills may not be your strengths. I've seen many women who start out feeling intimidated but who gradually become more confident with physicians and other personnel. They may have to force themselves at first to ask for what they want, but it gets easier each time they do.

Because your partner may be too sick or scared to put his concerns into words in the hospital, he may need you to do it for him. I remember one client who had major abdominal surgery. While recovering, he began to experience increased pain and was certain something was terribly wrong. However, when the doctor came by, he said nothing.

At that point, his wife stepped in to say: "He thinks he's backsliding because he has more pain today. Is that to be expected?" It turned out the problem was gas, which was actually a part of the recovery process and a good sign. Later, this husband thanked her for asking the question. Getting the facts made a huge psychological difference to him. All too often the truth is quite different from the fantasies in a patient's head.

Another good question at the hospital is "Why are you doing this?" Sometimes there isn't a good reason for yet another test or painful needle. You may never have taken the initiative before and feel reluctant (or just too tired) to do so. Yet you need to know what's going on. Your mate's well-being is at stake.

5. Consider comfort and convenience.

If you have a choice when selecting a hospital, realize that the best ones are usually teaching facilities affiliated with medical schools—but that doesn't mean all departments are created equal. This is another time when it helps to ask around and check online. *U.S. News & World Report* issues an annual ranking of the best hospitals in the country for sixteen different specialties. However, most patients go to local community hospitals. You can check out hospital performance data in some states online or ask knowledgeable medical professionals.

Is it worth traveling far away to get the best? It may be if: (a) the medical condition is unusual; (b) it's difficult to treat; or (c) successful intervention requires equipment or expertise that is available only in a handful of places. I know of one West Coast husband who was diagnosed with a complex brain tumor. His wife happened to see a TV show about a hospital in the Midwest that had pioneered surgery for this condition. Although it was inconvenient, time-consuming, and expensive to make the trip, the couple chose to have the surgery there. The operation was a complete success.

On the other hand, sometimes you may believe that the top hospital isn't the best choice if it's so far away that it means isolating you from your sources of support. There's comfort in remaining in familiar surroundings. This is one of those cases where practicalities, the chances of success, and insurance coverage should be considered.

6. See to his personal comfort.

Once your mate is in the hospital, try to see that he's as comfortable as possible. If he's in a semiprivate room and his roommate gives him headaches, request another room. Bring him an iPod if he loves music, or a book on tape if he likes to read. If the hospital will permit you to bring it, his own quilt from home can keep him feeling cozy and cared for. Place family photos on the bedside cabinet to help him feel connected.

Remember the importance of his dignity, and try to understand his reactions in the hospital. He wants to stay in control, to feel respected and masculine. If he insists on wearing his own robe and slippers from home instead of the hospital gown, you may want to retort, "Who cares what you're wearing? They've seen everything here." But since it may matter a great deal to him, bring them.

7. Know your rights if you're an unmarried partner.

Doctors and hospitals will protect the patient's privacy and won't give his medical information to anyone but next of kin—unless he tells them otherwise. This can be especially frustrating and problematic for significant others, who will be told, "I can only discuss his condition with a family member." The message is "You're an outsider."

If your partner hasn't already told his doctor it's okay to discuss all of his medical matters with you, it's time for him to do so. Otherwise, not only is he making your job more difficult, he is hurting himself. He should have a health care proxy and other documents in place that name you as his agent to make medical decisions if he is unable to. You may want to ask him to sign a health care proxy now if he doesn't already have one. You can also talk to the social worker, patient representative, or the hospital's legal department for guidance in such matters. (See pages 255–257 for information on relevant legal documents.) Preplanning helps. Keep in mind that in most states unmarried partners—whether heterosexual or homosexual—probably will not have the same status (or often get the same respect) as a spouse does.

STAYING ON COURSE

TODAY'S MEDICAL SYSTEM is like a labyrinth—an intricate combination of passages in which it is difficult to find your way. That's why it's important to educate and assert yourself in the system when necessary. Unless you're fortunate enough to have a physician or other health professional in the family to guide you, it's easy to get lost in the maze just when you and your mate are desperate for answers, help, and hope.

Reflections

- *Do your best to be present when your mate talks with the doctor. If that's not possible, delegate the job to a relative or friend who can be an effective surrogate.*

- *Keep asking questions until you get answers. Be willing to be a pest sometimes to get what your mate needs.*

- *Learn how to work the system. The more you know, the less frightened you'll be.*

- *Remember, healing often takes longer than you've been told. Hang in there.*

- *The hospital is a mysterious place, but you can learn about equipment and procedures and protect your mate's best interests.*

9

Work and Money: Protecting What You've Got

Your mate can't return to work for months after a serious accident or illness. Will his job be waiting? Or he's debilitated by medical treatment, yet continues to work. How understanding is his boss likely to be? Will health insurance cover the medical costs, or will you face a stack of bills? Will the demands of caring for him affect your own career? Or will you *have* to go to work when you wish to stay at home? His illness can shred the fabric of family security in more ways than one.

Such situations can be so upsetting that even the most organized people fall behind. You never anticipated that you'd have to handle so many responsibilities, and it's hard *not* to rush to the bottom line. Illness can wipe some families out financially. That's a fact.

On the other hand, I've watched clients set priorities, gather allies, and take advantage of available resources. They've learned how to work the system to get the benefits they're entitled to. Even in the worst circumstances, many find help that they didn't know existed or had never considered for themselves.

PROTECTING YOUR PARTNER'S
LIVELIHOOD WHEN HE'S EMPLOYED

IF YOUR PARTNER is too sick to work for a period of time, the challenge is to protect his job or keep his business up and running while containing your own overwhelming anxiety. You may find yourself dealing with his boss and other work-related contacts if he cannot. The burden can be backbreaking unless you cope with one issue at a time. The first priority is to notify his employer of what's going on and to enlist the maximum aid and support. Hopefully his employer will do everything possible to help you.

That was the case for Amelia and her husband, Greg, a Seattle landscape architect. After he suffered a stroke, his very generous boss allowed him to take off all the time he needed. As a result, Greg and Amelia never felt pressured and they knew his job was safe.

Although some companies are extraordinarily accommodating, others are more concerned with their balance sheet than with your problems. They may be less understanding especially if your mate is a relatively new employee. I know an administrator who accepted a position at ten a.m. on Wednesday and received the news that he had cancer at three p.m. the same day. Fortunately, the employer was a people-friendly nonprofit organization that was willing to hold his job for him while he completed a full course of treatment. A corporation or privately owned company might not be so obliging.

When your mate runs his own firm or business, his partners or employees may be the people who can hold down the fort until he's well enough to work (or work full time) again. You hope his partners will say, "Don't worry. We'll take care of everything till he's back on his feet."

It's far more difficult, however, if he works alone or has unique skills or talents. I remember Claire, a client whose husband had two major heart attacks. He was an attorney in a small practice. His one junior associate tried to keep the firm going. Claire hoped her husband would recover enough to go back at least part time, but that just wasn't possible. The firm foundered without him and closed.

Walking a Tightrope

During treatment and recuperation, try your best to keep appropriate people posted on your mate's progress. Along the way, it's wise to carefully consider what information you divulge and how. For example, at first you may not know how long your partner will be out (or even have nagging fears that he may never return to work). You need a confidant with whom you can discuss those anxieties. By all means talk to your sister or best friend if it helps. It's important to air your fears, not swallow them. But you may not want your doubts to reach his boss's ears at this point. You don't want to create uncertainty or box yourself in when the ultimate outcome is still unclear.

Great strides have been made in medicine in recent years. Twenty-five percent of stroke survivors recover with minor impairment, and another 10 percent recover completely, according to the National Institute of Neurological Disorders and Stroke. Most cancer patients go back to their jobs. Only one out of five cancer survivors is disabled or out of work five years after treatment, according to a Penn State study. Therefore, you may may find yourself walking the line between realistic decisions and the possibility of hope.

Fielding Inquiries from Others

You may also have to summon all your powers of diplomacy to handle concerned calls from your mate's clients, customers, or coworkers. One wife made it her mission to remain as positive and upbeat as possible after her husband had major surgery. When his accounts called to ask about his condition, she always used language such as, "He's coming along," rather than get into specifics. She called her responses "hold-them-at-bay tactics." When the doctor gave her a date for an expected return to work, she padded it, adding on a few weeks just in case there were complications or setbacks. "Truth comes in many forms," she says. "I did what I had to do to protect his livelihood."

Not without cost, however. She admits she paid a heavy emotional toll and found it exhausting to constantly parry inquiries and put a positive spin on what was happening. She felt like a press secretary. She told me:

I'll never forget my husband hanging over the toilet throwing up while I was on the phone with his best customer assuring him that my husband was in the shower and would call him back. I'd also say such things as, "He has a bad day here and there, which the doctor says is to be expected." I didn't want them to think, "He's too sick to come back. I'd better get someone else." I also know that rumors travel fast and far in the business world. Word gets around that can stop new business from coming to him in the future. It's a sticky situation.

You want to hear people say, "Concentrate on getting well. Don't worry. You'll always have our business." But is that true? How far will loyalty go? It can be a major worry.

To minimize disruption while your mate is out sick, you may also need the cooperation of coworkers who can assume some of his duties. This is the time to ask his most trusted colleagues to help. You don't have to do all of this yourself.

At the same time, you may also be in charge of damage control to protect his internal interests and ward off potential poachers at his company. My client Jenna recalls standing in intensive care and holding her husband's hand. The doctor, aware that the patient was a partner in a prestigious accounting firm, walked in to examine him. The physician spoke encouragingly and commented, "We don't want them going after the wounded whale." That one remark summed up her own fears that one of her mate's ambitious partners might try to undermine his position while he was flat on his back.

WHEN YOUR PARTNER CAN'T RETURN TO WORK

IT MAY BECOME apparent that a return to work just isn't possible. Your mate's job is now beyond his physical or mental capabilities. That happened to Amelia's husband, the landscape architect. His stroke caused cognitive and behavioral changes rather than physical disability. He often became agitated, confused, or simply stared ahead for periods of time. When he eventually tried to go back to work, he couldn't handle the job.

"His designs didn't work, but he thought everything was fine. Finally his boss called and told me it wasn't working out. He offered excellent severance pay, but it was a terrible financial blow," says Amelia. When the bad luck continued and Amelia subsequently lost her own job, the couple had to sell their large house and move into a small apartment. Never savers, their small nest egg didn't last long. Sometimes very painful decisions do have to be made.

YOUR OWN JOB PROBLEMS

IN THE MIDST of protecting his career, you may have your own work issues to deal with. Fifty-five percent of women who take care of an ill family member work full or part time. When you're employed, how do you handle your workload, child care (if you have kids), and take care of him, too? If you're like most people, you probably have to juggle, work late, take time off, or make other adjustments. In the case of a devastating diagnosis like Alzheimer's disease, you may work fewer hours or quit altogether. It's also common to turn down promotions or transfers because of caregiving demands. A woman has to be creative at a time like this to protect her interests.

Can Your Employer Help?

You aren't a magician. You can't take on the extra challenge of caring for your partner without help and understanding at work. Unfortunately, some people hesitate to reveal obligations at home. They fear the information will work against them, hindering chances for advancement or special projects. They worry people will say, "She's got too much going on to handle more responsibility." But it's usually unproductive to hide your situation. Instead, ask your boss or manager about flexible hours if you need them, or time off or long lunch hours to visit at the hospital or accompany your mate to tests. If you must miss a meeting or call home frequently, tell your employer why. An honest explanation makes more sense than allowing people to assume you're irresponsible or unreliable. Who knows? Your boss may have good suggestions, such as telecommuting or trading shifts.

If you ask, clients may work with you, too. Ruth, a freelance graphic artist, needed extra leeway when her husband had spinal surgery. Her accounts were sympathetic and supportive after she told them about the challenges she faced. They offered to help in any way they could, including postponing deadlines. People are usually empathetic when you're in a bind, but you can't expect them to guess what's going on.

When you need flexible hours and time off, it's best to negotiate them up front. The result may be more positive than you anticipate. I worked with one client who took time off to help her husband during his lengthy treatment for bladder cancer. Dedicated to her job, she put in extra effort to compensate for her absences. Her employer rewarded her with a big bonus and a raise. Although she constantly worried about her performance, she was doing a terrific job despite her burdens at home. It's easy to lose perspective about whether and how your caregiving duties will prejudice people against you at work. Sometimes a fresh, objective opinion from a trusted colleague can change your outlook.

Employee Assistance Programs

If you're lucky, your company may offer an employee assistance program that can help you. About 6 percent of American companies provide free services such as psychological and other counseling, referrals to legal assistance, and respite care for your mate, which allows you to take a break.

Claire, the woman whose husband's law practice closed, almost had an emotional breakdown before finally turning to help available at her workplace. "My husband had great difficulty tending to himself. I obsessed about his being home alone all day, but I had to keep working, because we needed the money and my health insurance. The stress finally got to me, so I took advantage of the free psychological counseling provided at my job. The counselor told me I had to go out and do things for myself, especially fun things." When you're in a tailspin, often you need someone else's permission to help you find time to play.

FOR SOME, WORK IS THERAPY

CLAIRE WOULD QUIT her job tomorrow if she could, but she has to work. Her income is essential to pay for increased heating bills and to hire plumbers and other outsiders to help her keep up with home repairs. "My husband used to fix the dishwasher and build the shelves I needed. That's all over now," she explains.

But we're all different. For other women, work is a lifesaver that provides structure and helps them go on when they feel they're drowning in their partners' needs. One wife loves getting out of the house to go to work—and the extra income, too. Her forty-five-year-old husband is in a wheelchair after a hit-and-run accident. She balances his needs and hers with creativity—she's employed in a computer programming job working from five a.m. to eleven a.m. "He sleeps in the morning. When I get home, he's just getting up. It works out well. If necessary, he can always call me by cell phone," she explains.

Florence, too, feels that her work saved her sanity on several occasions when her husband was seriously ill. "I get lost in it because it's challenging and I'm always learning something new, which is fuel for my soul. I also love interviewing people, researching, and networking with colleagues."

Of course, she's in a unique situation, because her children are grown, and her freelance career offers flexibility. She can set her own hours. Yet I know women in other occupations who echo her comments. Their jobs are stress reducers that enhance their sense of well-being. During times of trouble, immersion in their work becomes therapeutic and the one place in the midst of chaos where they can truly feed their self-esteem.

"Work helps me compartmentalize and focus on the problem at the moment," says Tanisha, a publicist who works at home. "But I'm lucky. I can be sitting at the computer at noon in my nightgown. If I had to get dressed up and be nice to everyone all day, I would have a hard time putting on a pretty face. In my case, I can go hours without talking to anyone. If you're a school-teacher or in sales, where you have to be 'on' and 'up' all the time, it's easier to get worn down. Annoying people can be *really* annoying when you're stressed." At such times, it becomes even more important to take care of yourself by taking a walk, going to the gym, or meeting a friend to chat and release pent-up feelings.

Be who you are. If work is a refuge for you, and you can afford it, it may make sense to pay someone else to help take care of your mate. Aides cost seven to fifteen dollars an hour or more, depending on your locale. If money is tight, consider a smart high school or college student who may be able to work odd hours and who probably wants extra cash. Post a notice on a school's bulletin board or call their employment center.

FINANCIAL GUIDANCE

"MY BIG ANXIETY is managing money," says Sherry, whose mate has been incapacitated by a rare neurological disease. She has three daughters to send to college. "Luke always took care of our investments even though I was in charge of the checkbook and paid all the bills. Fortunately, a stockbroker friend of our family has stepped in to manage a lot of it, so I don't feel so over-whelmed."

Even if you're well off, you may still need help with finances. Another client of mine, Marsha, had no experience with accounting, yet she had to assume responsibility for the finances of her mate's small company during his prolonged illness. She felt so afraid of what she didn't know that her eyes glazed over at the numbers. Her solution: she asked a friend to sit with her while she looked at her husband's company's balance sheet. Just having that support gave her the strength to begin to deal with the task before her. In fact, Marsha grew into a pretty good businesswoman. She discovered a talent she never thought she had.

HELPFUL INTERNET ADDRESSES FOR MONEY AND INSURANCE CONCERNS

MANY ONLINE sites, including some dedicated specifically to care-givers, provide information on finances and insurance, such as www.familycaregiving101.org/help/financial.cfm and www.strength forcaring.com (click "money" and "insurance").

Here are some other helpful Web sites:

- **www.benefitscheckup.org:** This is a National Council on Aging site for people fifty-five and older.
- **www.GovBenefits.gov:** Offers information on benefits available for both younger and older people and helps you determine your eligibility.
- **www.ssa.gov:** Information on two federal Social Security Administration disability programs. Social Security Disability Insurance (SSDI) pays when your mate cannot work. Social Security Supplemental Insurance (SSI) covers very low-income individuals of any age who are blind or disabled.

You may need help from your husband's office (or your own); your accountant, if you have one; your sister who has an account-ing degree; or the uncle who has always been a good financial adviser. You want all the information and guidance you can get as early as you can—before you're flailing around looking for a life preserver.

Health insurance may not pay for every test or scan. Copayments tend to add up, no matter what your coverage. Uncovered medications or home care, medical supplies, and equipment cost money. Sadly, you can have health insurance and still get into debt.

Many disease-specific organizations, such as the National Kidney Foundation and CancerCare, can provide information or certain types of financial assistance. Some can help with medical bills, assist with child care and other costs, steer you to grants and other possibilities, and may provide vocational rehabilitation.

Social workers at the hospital can locate financial resources and help with entitlements such as Medicaid. Your place of worship may offer financial aid, and some drug companies offer free medications to those who cannot afford them (call the Partnership for Prescription Assistance at 800-762-4636 for a directory of programs).

SEVEN STEPS TO HOLDING IT ALL TOGETHER

IF YOUR MATE is incapacitated for more than a brief period, the finances of your entire family may be on shaky ground. Depending on health insurance and the extent of employer goodwill, financial hardship may be a distinct possibility. Here's how to protect your mate's position (and your own, if you are employed) and get assistance:

1. **Follow a to-do list for his job.**
    To protect your mate and minimize workplace disruption while he's out, contact his boss or company or partners quickly to fill them in on what has happened. Then prioritize:

    - Find out how much medical leave and paid vacation he is entitled to.

    - Check the details of his health insurance plan (or yours, if you have the coverage) to find out what is and isn't covered. Provisions can vary, and there may be deadlines for ordering certain services or medical equipment.

■ If he has to leave his job, be aware that COBRA (Consolidated Omnibus Budget Reconciliation Act), a federal law, permits him to continue employer health insurance coverage for eighteen to thirty-six months, depending on the circumstances. However, he, not his employer, must pay for it.

■ Find out if he is eligible for disability benefits. If so, apply for them quickly; it takes time for payments to start arriving in the mailbox. Disability insurance pays if he is unable to work due to illness or injury. Payment is usually 60 to 70 percent of gross income. If your mate has his own private disability plan, payments vary.

His company's human resources or personnel department may be the place to go for information on all of the above, and may offer other support. Check with your insurance agent for information on private disability insurance.

2. Know his rights and yours.

In a way, there's never been a better time to confront disability. Companies don't want to be sued. The Americans with Disabilities Act (ADA) protects your mate from job discrimination if he works for a company with more than fifteen people. The law requires employers to make "reasonable accommodations" for him to get his job done, such as flexible hours or a wheelchair-friendly work space.

To Tell or Not to Tell About the Disease can be a Complex Question. Although we've come a long way, now that people such as the former attorney general Janet Reno and the actor Michael J. Fox have gone public with their diagnoses, it isn't far enough. Severe illness is still considered shameful by some people in our society, and some people with multiple sclerosis and Parkinson's disease hide the information because they're afraid they'll lose their jobs. Be aware, however, that the ADA will protect your mate *only* if he speaks up. This is one of those times to get legal advice, as well as counsel from wise people around you, rather than make the decision alone.

You've Got a Law, Too. If you work for a company with fifty or more employees and must tend to a severely ill family member, the Family Medical Leave Act gives you the right to an unpaid leave of absence of up to twelve weeks (with benefits) in a twelve-month period. Note that the federal law does not include unmarried partners in its definition of "spouse." However, several state laws do.

Unmarried partners' rights generally differ from state to state. I always advise clients to check out local laws. To make sure that you can access funds for your partner's care if he is incapacitated, there are simple precautions the two of you can take, such as putting both names on a bank account, investments, or an apartment lease. It's a matter of trust, and couples must weigh the positives and negatives of taking such steps.

3. **Make decisions with him if you can.**

When his condition permits, talk to your mate about how to handle job-related and financial matters, and try to understand his point of view. If he is disabled in some way, does he want to work if he can? How do you feel about that?

Allison was a stay-at-home mom whose working husband was increasingly debilitated by cancer treatment. She insisted, "I want you to stop working and stay home. I'll get a job." Fortunately, she was in a caregiver support group that shared emotional support and practical information. The group told her, "It's a great sentiment, but you need to discuss it more fully with your husband. There may be reasons he wants to maintain a connection with work. Also, it could be more stressful for him to stay home, take care of the kids, and do household tasks he's not accustomed to doing."

Allison got specific advice on how to talk with her husband and heard ideas from others who had been through similar situations. They advised her first to think through what she wanted to say, then sit down and have a discussion with him so that he could voice his own perspective. They told her, "This isn't something you get a script for. You're not a failure." She went home with a sense of hope.

A post-treatment support group may be helpful for your partner in such a situation. Members can help him deal with the effects of treatment, such as side effects, dietary changes, and psychosocial adjustments if he can't work. In some cases, adjustments in the way he handles his job may be all that is needed.

4. Help him look at other work options, if necessary.

If it is no longer possible for your partner to do his job, perhaps he can perform in another capacity where his particular disability is not an issue. For example, many airlines will offer a desk job to a pilot or flight attendant who has been grounded due to disability.

If he's in the construction industry but can no longer

lift heavy loads after a heart attack, can he supervise? He may not be able to travel across the country to see customers, but maybe he can handle telephone sales or even work from home. If permanent disability stops him from working full time, perhaps a part-time schedule is feasible. And sometimes choices can change. A friend of mine, a disabled physician, retired and became a writer. Then he missed working with people and started up a part-time practice again.

Some disease-specific organizations, such as the American Stroke Association, offer information on retraining for another kind of work if that is feasible, or may even help him find another job. Some stroke survivors have launched their own businesses. New opportunities may be found.

5. **Take advantage of employee assistance programs for caregivers.**

These programs tend to be underutilized. People don't know about them, feel that what's going on at home is private, or assume that if word gets out about their responsibilities, it will look bad, hurt performance ratings, or even get them fired. Yet you can't get help unless you ask.

Some companies subsidize adult day care or emergency home care for an ill family member. It's worth it to the organization to pay an outside provider rather than have you take time off. Some employers allow workers to donate vacation time to others who have used up their allotment and need more time off to care for a sick family member.

6. **Balance work and caregiving.**

Try to make phone calls or schedule your partner's doctors' appointments during your lunch hour. When you have an important business event you can't miss, you can also ask your family, friends, or volunteers from your community or place of worship to help you out and monitor your mate, especially if you give them plenty of advance notice.

Reciprocate help from coworkers when you can. Offer to pitch in when they're overwhelmed, and remember the words "Thank you." It means a lot to people to know that they're appreciated. If the help is ongoing, consider sending a thank-you note saying something like, "What would I do without you?" or "You're a lifesaver." If you prefer, send a card or a small gift.

A caregiver support group can give you perspective on work decisions. Sometimes people leave jobs to care for their mates and take on financial risk or too much change and wear themselves out. Group members challenge one another or offer advice in such situations, such as, "Don't you think you need some help? What about day care? I put my husband in day care, and that opened up time for me. What about four hours a day?"

If someone says, "I can't do that to my husband" or "He'll reject my having help to take care of him," members can break through some of the denial and resistance to getting help. Don't force yourself into a mold that doesn't suit you unless you have no choice.

7. Get everyone involved.

"I have the financial support of my husband's family, which has made all the difference. They provided my husband with home health care and have taken care of me since I've become disabled myself," says Fran. In fact, I've seen many cases where families help out financially. A relative may pay the mortgage and bills until disability payments come through or provide monthly stipends to help make ends meet—or simply send over a cleaning service once a week.

Help can arrive in other ways, too. I think of one notable case where a well-loved orthopedist was dying of ALS (Lou Gehrig's disease) over a very long period of time. Patients and their families, colleagues, and friends—the entire community—responded to his tragedy by organizing an annual walkathon to raise money for his family's support. His wife and children survived financially in part because of this help.

Sometimes people volunteer such assistance on their own. Sometimes they don't, and you may have to be the creative one and suggest the idea. I know how difficult it is to request what may seem like charity. But when your family's survival is at stake, there is nothing to be ashamed of. Hard as it may be, reach out.

HANDLING THE FALLOUT

IF IT'S ANY comfort, the impact of a partner's illness on work has certain universal qualities, no matter what the position. For example, each year an estimated twenty-two CEOs of S&P 500 companies suffer life-threatening health problems that substantially affect their ability to do their jobs, according to the *Wall Street Journal.* They have heart attacks and cancer just like everyone else, and often leave their companies unprepared for their incapacitation.

Of course their families are unlikely to have the same financial worries you do. Medical expenses are at the root of almost half of personal bankruptcies in this country. The financial burden for many families can be crushing. But don't panic. Remember, often there are resources at the workplace, in the community, and in the family that can help. Use them.

Reflections

- *The key word is "early." Tell your partner's boss about his illness early; apply for disability early. It takes a long time to get payments rolling.*

- *Talk to your boss if you're employed. It's stressful and usually unproductive to hide your situation.*

- *Know the laws that protect your partner (and you).*

- *Work together with your partner if his condition permits.*

- *Take it one issue at a time to get through this.*

PART THREE

Taking Care of
Your Relationship

10

The Power of
Transformational Love

Most couples can get through the good times in life. It's during the bad times that the bond between you is tested. This is a rough road you're on, full of potholes and unexpected turns that can stress the strongest relationships and conspire to distance the two of you. The task is to prevent that from happening. I understand how difficult it is to struggle with your mate's serious illness and tend to your relationship at the same time. But I'm going to help you find ways to protect the closeness you've got, build on that foundation, and draw strength from each other.

What pulls you through the ordeal is commitment. This is what your vow "for better or worse" really means. Along with commitment comes the possibility of a little-explored concept known as *transformational love*. The question you face is: Can the experience of illness become an opportunity to discover this new kind and depth of love? Can you rise to the challenge with a strength that you may not have realized was in you? It's a test of character, and you may not know what you're made of until you're faced with a catastrophe.

WHAT IS TRANSFORMATIONAL LOVE?

WHEN I TALK about transformational love, I refer to deep, enduring love—a connection between two people that usually goes far beyond anything they have experienced before. Most of us *think* we know what that love is, but we don't really understand its full meaning until disaster strikes and we feel heartache and pain. It is then that you have the opportunity to peel away layers of your relationship to find the core of what really matters: survival and sustaining your deep connection to each other.

Transformational love is a process, and it occurs in ways you may not have understood before. All that you may have thought was important before your partner's illness—success, making more money, a bigger house, a better car—falls aside. What counts is the bond between you. The challenge is to support that bond to withstand forces you can't always control. This can be a life-changing experience, one that brings new meaning and maturity to your relationship and lasts forever. Transformational love may sound like an illusion, an impossible ideal. But it is not.

Florence experienced this process during the course of her husband's illnesses. She describes it this way: "I discovered what love really is. It's feeling your heart break when he's hurting or struggling. It's bursting with pride when he finds the courage to pick himself up and go on after a setback knocks him down. It's holding your tongue and listening as he searches for the best treatment option instead of rushing in to fill the void of uncertainty. It's putting your own anxiety aside for the greater good—his."

Florence found within herself a generosity and a reservoir of courage that continually surprised her. "I'm very proud of myself, but I had no idea what I was capable of at the beginning. I grew from a trembling 'girl' to an effective adult woman."

At a time when your plans, your expectations, and your future may seem to be crumbling, you either drown in desperation and despair, or you ride the waves and prevail. But you don't ever remain the same. If you survive, you have the chance to set new priorities and focus on the fact that you and your partner have different needs. In order to get through this, his needs must come first when appropriate and necessary, but you must also find ways to live your own life—to balance generosity with self-preservation.

That is transformational love. It involves a collaborative effort between you and your partner. During many years of practice, I have watched people pass through the process, and I have seen this special kind of love grow and develop. It is infinitely richer than anything they've felt before. Couples who are willing to learn from the illness they've faced together relate the same experience. My aim is to show you that in spite of what can be a searing struggle, you *can* reach for that growth and realize it together. You begin by understanding that certain prerequisites make transformational love possible.

EXPERIENCING YOUR EMOTIONAL PAIN

WHEN THE MAN you love is ill, you're going to feel emotions at times that are unwanted and unpleasant, such as fear, sadness, guilt, perhaps even hate. Sometimes you may wish the ordeal were over with—possibly even that your partner would die. Most people are afraid to acknowledge such thoughts and feelings. They think they are unacceptable. They tend to hide or deny them to make them disappear. Instead these feelings may emerge in destructive ways, such as depression or physical symptoms.

Maybe you're afraid to feel sad that life may never be the same. It's common to assume that if you feel an intense emotion, you will have to *act* on it. You might want to run away. In fact, however, the feeling *can* be contained. Keep in mind that thoughts and feelings are just that—thoughts and feelings. They won't destroy you and don't make you a shameful wife or partner; they're part of being human. Uncomfortable emotions are one of the prices you pay for a loving relationship during serious illness. It's just plain hard work.

Don't be afraid to feel all of your sorrow. It is only when you experience the depth of your pain that you can get past it and move on. When you want to sob in despair, it helps to surrender to it. If you always swallow your tears, it's difficult to heal, and your feelings build up. They need an outlet; the energy has to go somewhere. Cry when you must, and you cleanse yourself. Then you're free to go on and cope. You may think an always strong facade will save you from falling apart, when in fact buried feelings can show through on your face or cause some other part of your body to give way.

Equally important, the ability to feel painful emotions helps open the door to feeling *positive* emotions. It is difficult to feel the deepest love unless you've also experienced your deepest despair. My client Joan found herself thinking, "I love my husband fiercely." Such a statement would never have occurred to her before he got sick. "I'd never have felt that kind of love if we hadn't looked death in the eye and gone through hell together," she told me. "I wouldn't have known what the words meant."

ACKNOWLEDGING LOSSES

ACKNOWLEDGING YOUR LOSSES is another requirement for the process of transformational love. Depending on the nature of your partner's condition, serious illness always involves losses. Some of them may be enormous. The goal is to identify your losses clearly, hold them to the light, and begin the process of mourning them one at a time. That's how you work them through. The mystery and power of loss dissolves. It's when your thinking is muddied that your situation seems insurmountable.

Your own losses may involve some or all of the following:

Loss: Peace of mind

Many women view the men they love as pillars to lean on—strong and invulnerable. A serious illness shatters that perception forever. Joan found that statistics were the worst part when her husband had to undergo an extended and risky treatment. "They told us that 35 percent of people who go through this die. That was terrifying to contemplate," she recalls.

Even if he has recovered from a stroke or heart attack—or the cancer hasn't recurred—the fallout from the original event often lingers years later. You may never feel crisis-free again. Somewhere deep down you live with the worry that another bout of illness may be just around the corner. In chronic conditions such as Crohn's disease or arthritis, there may be good days (or weeks) and bad ones that unsettle your life and make planning ahead difficult.

No, you can't return to the days when serious illness was something that happened to other people. It's normal to vent and obsess about what was and what may be. But ultimately you do have to smell the roses, even if they have thorns.

Loss: He's not the man he used to be

Even if your mate has been able to resume a relatively normal life, he may not be able to do some of the things he used to. Maybe you have to open the car door for *him*. Perhaps he once was a dapper dresser and the life of the party but no longer has the energy. Or he used to be so independent, and now he calls you sixteen times a day at your office.

You may find it painful to see a strong man become needy.

Your heart aches as you watch him struggle down the stairs. Once you acknowledge those feelings, you can focus on all that he is *now*. One man lost fifty pounds during his illness. His wife Norma told me:

> He's a bag of bones, and of course it bothers me. But I've also realized my attraction to him isn't based on how he looks. He's a hero after what he's dragged himself through. And he's still the man I can turn to for advice about my job and family problems. His wisdom, his know-how, his good sense bring me such security. He has an honesty and ability to help me cut through to the core of a problem.
>
> I look at other men, and none of them measures up to him. We were lying on the couch in the living room yesterday, and I felt such love for him. I was glad for him to be stretched out beside me, holding me; just that comforts me.

The essence of who your partner is usually remains, or may even have grown in new ways. Sometimes there is actually more to love.

Loss: Lifestyle changes

You may not be able to do the things you used to do. Your social life as a couple may dwindle, because you can't go out as much together. Some people stop inviting you to dinners, because you can't reciprocate. You no longer entertain at home, because you never know how he's going to feel ahead of time. Maybe you can't take vacations in exotic places, because you want to be close to good medical care, or driving trips are too exhausting for him, or your finances won't permit it. Perhaps it seems your life consists of running from one doctor's appointment to another.

Norma softens the blow of a constricting social life by taking her husband in his wheelchair on walks, to local restaurants, and to movies. They often read books or watch TV together in the same room. Just feeling each other's presence is comforting intimacy.

Loss: Role reversals

If your mate was the one who always took charge of things, and you like it that way, his illness can put a strain on your marriage. You may want to be a pampered woman—and that may no longer be possible. "I depended on him. He was so strong," you remind yourself. Now *you're* dealing with the insurance agent and the accountant, and you hate it. Or he can't drive and you're the chauffeur. Or he doesn't *want* to take care of home-maintenance chores anymore. He expects you to call the plumber and arrange for the lawn to be mowed—and you've already got enough to do. Or you may like being a working woman, but you must stay home to take care of him.

A big roadblock to transformational love can be resistance to asking for help, which can breed anger toward (and distance from) your partner and cause anxiety or depression in you. Sometimes help isn't available and you may have to do what you don't like. Too often, however, women accept that there is no other way except feeling trapped and doing everything themselves, when that isn't true. You can learn when to say no and prioritize to avoid your own personal prison.

REASSESSING WHY YOU'RE TOGETHER

ANOTHER PART OF the process of transformational love is reexamining the reasons you and your partner are together and then making adjustments. This is a time when you confront the big issues honestly: Are you together now because you love each other—or for other honorable reasons, such as shared history, the children you raised, an indefinable bond? Are there economic, family, or religious considerations? For Joan, the answer is, "My husband knows how to treat a woman. To him, I'm a princess. I love him so much."

What does your partner bring to the relationship? Does he take care of you emotionally, despite the fact that he tires easily or walks with a cane or can't work anymore? Does he provide companionship even if he spends most of his time in bed? Family and financial security? Practical knowledge? A loving heart?

Nicole, forced to become the sole wage earner after her husband was severely injured, wants to retire and move near her sister, but she hasn't done anything about it, because *she* will have to handle the arrangements. "It's so hard to make all the decisions myself," she says. Yet she also keeps in mind what her husband *does* do.

"He nourishes me in the ways that he can. He always tells people he'd be dead without me. If I hadn't been at the hospital, he wouldn't have eaten. He is still able to cook and has a hot meal waiting for me when I come home from work. I am lucky," she adds.

Over time this couple has worked out their role reversal. As much as living near her sister might make her life easier, what she's got is working well enough for now.

Maybe your partner can't attend your friend's New Year's Eve party, but can you feel joy in the children you share? Can you be glad knowing that no one else in the world understands the love and pride you feel in your kids—that he feels it, too? These are the precious intangibles of life.

No matter how much you love your mate, there may be times when you ask yourself, "Is it worth it?" Whether or not you have doubts about the answer, it's helpful to formulate an internal emotional checklist, as the women just mentioned have done.

Surely one of the cruelest losses occurs when illness or injury affects his cognitive ability. "Who he is" may be gone. He may not want (or be able) to listen to your troubles. You have to find friends for that, and other outlets, such as a therapist or a support group. Sometimes you can only take one day at a time. If your faith is a source of comfort, embrace it for spiritual solace.

If he no longer knows who you are, at some point you may think, "I don't want to stay." This is a normal feeling. Give yourself permission to have it. The decision is whether you act on it. Do you hang in there? Do you have an affair? Do you leave? Or do you seek another path and build supportive communities at your place of worship or elsewhere to help you get through this?

Remember, you're making a moral and ethical choice. You're rising to a better part of yourself to become a person you didn't even know you wanted to be. Isabel , who has cared for years for a husband with dementia, feels this way: "It's not a prison sentence. Life is a series of choices. Every day has to be a choice. Otherwise it *is* a sentence, and you feel used and resentful and do a real number on the relationship."

REWORKING YOUR DREAMS

DREAMS MAY BE seen as wishes and hopes. When your partner's condition dashes your dreams, it can change your expectations, and you may experience new emotions. Although rituals exist to help you cope with the loss of a loved one, none are available to help bury your dreams. Maybe you thought you'd have children and live happily ever after. Now children may not be possible. Or you expected you'd have a partner to have fun with. Now that's out of the question. You thought you'd enjoy retirement, traveling, and visiting your grandchildren, but it's too difficult. You stay home. You thought you'd grow old and sit on the porch in rockers together. Instead you may be alone.

Sometimes lost dreams are smaller, but special to you nonetheless. Maybe you wanted to renovate your home—remodel your kitchen or add a den or office. Now the money has to go for an aide or medical expenses. You're going to have to live with what you've got or even scale back. It can be painful to give up your original dreams. The challenge is to reach out to others, change your attitude, and reshape your expectations.

Can you appreciate what you've got? Grace recalls all the complications that her husband suffered during a long recuperation from cancer surgery. When he finally started feeling a little better, Grace was very happy that they could walk around the corner and eat dinner at a coffee shop on Saturday night after weeks of being housebound. "It was one of our 'little triumphs.' I used to need so much more—the theater or the latest trendy restaurant. Now what counted were the ability to go out— anywhere at all—and a change of scenery. A glass of cheap wine and a tuna fish platter looked awfully good to me," she says. Part of transformational love means accepting the reality of your partner's condition but also realizing that there is a lot of life left in him and in your relationship.

SOME MARRIAGES DON'T REACH THE GOAL

NOT EVERYONE ACHIEVES transformational love, nor does everyone even want to try. There are couples who survive illness and stay together out of inertia or fear of being alone. In other cases, the healthy spouse stays in part to repay a debt. "I'm diabetic. When I had an operation the year before his diagnosis, and my leg got infected, he took care of me," explains one woman.

Edith had Parkinson's disease when she married. Her husband knew and accepted the challenges ahead. "I went through two years of nothing but crying, and he was so good to me. I felt my life was over, but he was a saint. Now he's sick. How can I not do the same for him?" she asks.

Several years ago, Edith's husband, a New Hampshire financial consultant, was diagnosed with a rare disease. "Finally, a new medication came out that worked like a miracle. He's better, but it's horrible. When he was in bed, I knew he'd be there. Now that he's partly well, we can't plan anything. He can seem fine and we'll arrange to go to the mall. Then at two p.m. he says, 'I can't go. I have to go to bed.' This whole pattern is very lonely for me. I sit home evening after evening by myself," says Edith.

"I've lost the person who can stand on ladders and change lightbulbs and was healthy when I wasn't. I've lost the personal attraction between us. I spend a lot of time saying 'this isn't what I signed up for,' but it wasn't what he signed up for, either, so I feel guilty. I'm not the most patient person in the world when he goes to bed at odd times. But how can I be a bitch about it, which I feel I am."

Some people feel as though caregiving has wrung them dry, especially if they want to be taken care of themselves. They may get stuck in their losses, unable to process them and move on.

Edith stays in her marriage, but some relationships fall apart and the healthy spouse leaves. You may not have the same ties that bind if you've been together a relatively short time and don't have children together. If your relationship was wobbly to begin with, illness may magnify profound, unresolved issues between you, such as his alcoholism or your jealousy of his relationship with his family. Some people believe the reasons to leave far outweigh the reasons to stay and aren't willing to take on the difficult challenge of working problems out.

For example, Kitty couldn't cope with the personality changes and bizarre behavior caused by her husband's condition. "He was not the same person. I married a very vital man with high standards, who eroded into a victim who can't or won't do anything to help himself. He stopped caring about grooming or even going to the bathroom. He didn't care that his pants were soiled." After he lost his job in the computer industry, he began drinking heavily.

They separated when Kitty felt she had to leave to avoid sinking into despair. He now lives in a Dallas condo with dishes piled up in the sink and bills left unpaid. His neighbors complain that he stands on the balcony in his underwear, watching people with binoculars.

Kitty, who is building a career as a commercial real estate broker, speaks to him every day on the phone and occasionally visits. He constantly professes his love for her. The jury is still out on whether this marriage will survive. She can't bring herself to file for divorce. "Our family said, 'How could she do such a thing?' But I was drowning. Why should I suffer? Yet I feel guilty at the same time," she says. It's a hard decision. I've seen people obsess endlessly before finally taking that step.

Kitty is one of those people who are caught between trying to do the right thing and surviving themselves. For her, as for many women, the world of "for better, for worse" exists in a gray area where it is difficult to maneuver.

Other Relationships Last Beyond Legal Limits

On the other hand, sometimes there are ties that even divorce does not cast asunder. The bond to a former mate can remain surprisingly strong or resurface when illness strikes. Some divorced spouses return to take care of their sick or dying exes. Their motivations include compassion, history, friendship, children, and even love. Long after the split, the memory of what was and a personal moral compass still matter. A woman I know returned to take care of her children's dying father twenty years after they had divorced. He was her first love, and she never lost her feelings for family.

Others choose alternative courses. One woman was in the midst of a divorce when her husband was diagnosed with esophageal cancer. She stayed to care for him until the end. At the same time, she maintained a significant loving relationship with a man she eventually married. Lenore, whose husband had Alzheimer's disease, fell in love with another man. She divorced her husband with the understanding that she and her new mate would live with and care for her first husband. Not everyone would feel comfortable with these choices or find them moral. For others, they are solutions in painful circumstances.

THE SIX-STEP PATH TOWARD TRANSFORMATIONAL LOVE

IT ISN'T EASY to find a deeper connection with your man in the face of serious illness. Sometimes you have to fight for it. Here's how to start moving in the right direction:

1. Mourn your losses.

Depending on the diagnosis or situation, the nature of losses varies. The first step in dealing with your own losses is to name them—and even list them on a sheet of paper. This breaks loss down into small pieces that can be managed one at a time. You can begin to talk about your losses—sometimes with your partner, sometimes with others. The idea is to express your denial, anger, and sadness. Then you have a better chance to work through these feelings and eventually come to a place of acceptance of what is. You can begin to solve problems and avoid getting stuck.

Grace finally reached acceptance when she was able to admit to herself, "I don't know if we'll ever get our life back." Then she could begin to think in terms of "What can we do to live as full a life as possible?"

There are almost always ways to make your life better. That doesn't mean you can "fix" his medical condition, but you *can* think about how to make adjustments and maximize the positives in your life.

2. Put losses in perspective.

When you're panicked, it's natural to jump to cata-clysmic conclusions. You may think, "Our life is over," which sets up a situation that is impossible to deal with. Instead, you can break it down to specifics, such as, "We can't go to museums or take long walks in the park any-more." This way you're looking at a particular problem and can explore possible options. Perhaps a wheelchair would work—or, if necessary, visiting a museum with a friend.

Maybe a nicely furnished home has always been important to you, and now your partner's medical equip-ment makes your house seem like a hospital. A hospital bed takes over the bedroom. You walk in the door after work, and the first thing you see is his walker. You may think, "My home has been hijacked," and feel your refuge is gone. Yet there are ways to minimize disrup-tion. The home care department at the hospital may have some ideas. Members of a caregiver support group may have tips on how they managed. Even the customer serv-ice department of the equipment manufacturer (or the delivery people) may be helpful.

Be realistic about whether the loss is temporary or per-manent. In a long recovery there's a tendency to think, "He'll never get out of that wheelchair." That may not be true. Physical rehabilitation takes time. It helps to talk with the doctor or physical therapy team about what is and isn't realistic.

3. Learn to compartmentalize.

Put your worries about another potential disaster aside so that they don't stop you from enjoying what you can today. Obsessing won't prepare you for the next episode, but it will destroy your pleasure in life right now. Experience today, not what might happen next month or next year. Live in the moment with preparation. Make sure your mate has the pills he needs, and keep his doctors' phone numbers handy for emergencies, but live your life.

4. Get help for role reversals.

It doesn't have to take a CPA to handle your finances if you hate doing it. A trusted friend or relative, or someone from your place of worship, might be happy to earn extra money by handling such a task for you (or be willing to do it gratis). People say, "I won't give them my checkbook," but you have to be flexible to get the help you need to deal with home repairs or other issues. Stubbornness only ensures that your resentment will grow.

Brainstorm with friends, too, asking for specific advice, such as, "What can I do about food shopping when I can't leave him alone?" Someone with a fresh perspective may suggest an idea you never thought of before, such as ordering groceries online. Friends may volunteer to shop for you (or to stay with him while you get out of the house for a while and go to the supermarket yourself).

5. Realize that you're vulnerable.

A helper who gets no sleep is like the mother of a newborn—exhausted and drained. If a male friend says, "Margaret, sweetie, I love your husband, but you're running yourself ragged. Let me take you out to dinner," he suddenly seems like a knight on a white horse. Before you know it, you can wind up in bed with him. It happens. He's paying attention to your needs at a time when you're feeling depleted and lonely.

I've found that some people have a moral or religious base that sustains them and helps them resist temptation. They live in a world of defined morality. The thought of seeking solace outside of the marriage bed remains a foreign concept to them. For others, the choice to act or not act is based on the consequences. You need to ask yourself: "Is this what I really want in view of the costs? A kiss or more may seem like a wonderful thing to do tonight, but how will I feel about myself tomorrow morning?"

One way to tell if your action is something you'll regret later is to ask yourself, "How would I feel if this extramarital relationship became known?" If you'd feel ashamed, you want to think hard about it. Think about short-term gains that may cause you long-term pain. The last thing you need at this time is more worry.

You're hanging in with your partner for a reason. You have to decide whether you are making a sacrifice because you're a martyr, or if it's a moral and ethical choice for the good of all, one that is to be admired.

6. Treat your relationship like a treasure hunt.

In any relationship, hunt for the gifts you share, which can become too easy to forget. During illness, especially long-term illness, the clues to the treasure may take time to decipher. You may forget the way your partner makes you smile or the comfort he gives you at the end of the day, because he's a different person now. The gifts may even change. You may now see in him strength, persistence, and a willingness to keep going in spite of depression—and thus feel a new respect for him.

When Grace tried the hunt, she realized how her husband had always helped her through difficult decisions. "When I had to move my mother from assisted living into a nursing home, he forced me to face my ambivalence. When our son wanted to be a waiter after college, he reassured me that it didn't make him a bum—that he just needed time to figure out what he wanted to do. Of course he was right," she says.

As you care for your mate, pay attention to what you receive for all your efforts—his help, his love, his presence. Says one woman whose husband has slowly progressed to being housebound, "It isn't fun, but it beats being alone. At least I have him."

STAYING THE COURSE

GOING THROUGH A significant illness is like riding a roller coaster: there are ups and downs. Both of you experience periods of despair, denial, and feeling overwhelmed. It takes time for the process of transformational love to develop. There are setbacks when you may feel that achieving such love is an impossible goal. On such occasions, remember that the setbacks are only bumps. What sustains you is hope—*realistic* hope, the belief that this journey will take you to a better place regardless of the medical outcome. It can. I've seen it happen.

In her essay "The Power of Love to Transform and Heal," in the book *This I Believe,* Jackie Lantry writes, "I believe in the ingredients of love, the elements from which it is made. . . . Love is primal. It is comprised of compassion, care, security and a leap of faith. I believe in the power of love to transform." So do I.

Reflections

- *Transformational love is possible.*

- *Identify your losses and mourn them.*

- *Revisit the reasons you and your partner are together.*

- *Balance generosity with self-preservation.*

- *Remember, you're making a moral and ethical decision.*

11

Staying Close

You're only human. The stress of your mate's illness can undermine your sense of security and self-esteem and create tensions in your marriage. Under the strain, sometimes you manage to rise to the occasion and function well enough. Sometimes you don't. You may regress and fall back into old, destructive patterns like whining, complaining, or blaming that can drive the two of you apart. It helps to build in mechanisms that soften the blows to your confidence and strengthen the bond between you at the same time.

BUILDING INTIMACY

AS YOU RESET priorities to meet the demands of your partner's illness, protecting the intimacy between you is paramount and becomes a path to transformational love. Intimacy allows both of you to tackle what you must discuss—pragmatic decisions regarding medical treatment, work, or housing choices, as well as issues of daily life involving family, children, and the two of you as a couple. Intimacy is an elusive concept that can be difficult to define. It involves sharing each other's innermost selves and understanding and accepting each other's strengths and weaknesses. Intimacy in a relationship is almost always expressed through the couple's style of verbal and nonverbal communication, including looks, touches, and honest words.

Levels of intimacy vary widely in marriages. In some, partners lead separate lives with little emotional sharing; at the other end of the spectrum, they share every activity and thought. For most couples, the healthiest level of intimacy is somewhere in between—a balance of two separate people who can still remain closely connected to each other. During the process of transformational love, as you and your partner face the uncertainties of the future together, you will have the opportunity to become more intimate in new ways. Because you're in new territory, you may feel uncomfortable at first.

Many people put off deeper intimacy, even when health isn't an issue, because it's frightening to bare heart and soul to someone else and risk being vulnerable. When illness intrudes, it's an extra challenge that can pull a couple apart at a time when it's more important than ever to work together and support each other.

It is often difficult to overcome resistance to intimacy, but now there is no time to waste. This is an opportunity to learn that you can accept a greater level of closeness than you thought possible. The illusion that distance makes you safe and you can run away from what you have to deal with is just that—an illusion.

EXPANDING COMMUNICATION SKILLS

APPROPRIATE HONESTY IS the glue of intimacy. Even if you and your partner aren't the best communicators, you can take this chance to stretch and open up to each other as you deal with your most important challenges. In my years of practice, I've found that many couples don't really know how to talk to each other intimately. They often make tremendous progress when they learn specific strategies and exact words to use.

For example, men sometimes view talking about their illness as a sign of weakness. Because our society glorifies macho behavior, your mate may keep his fears and other feelings to himself rather than share them with you. As a woman, you face barriers to communication, too. You may hesitate to admit your own feelings because you feel too scared or don't want to burden him. This can create distance between you, which can be the beginning of a dead relationship. Usually, when communication and connection stop, so does sex. Fortunately, there are ways to prevent or halt this downward spiral.

THE HUSBAND MANUAL

I ONCE WORKED with a couple I'll call Dan and Rose, who had to deal with his diagnosis of prostate cancer. Although they loved each other deeply, they constantly squabbled as they struggled with treatment decisions and other complex issues. Every day, Rose would hand Dan his pills and bark, "Take your meds," as if she were talking to the kids. Her orders compounded Dan's anger at his own helplessness, and he'd react by lashing out at her. Instead of pulling together to reason and support each other, they were driving a wedge in their relationship. The household tension started to affect their three children. That's when they came to me.

In the course of his work in therapy, Dan became more insightful and creative. One day he pulled out a notebook featuring a to-do list for Rose. It detailed what he wanted her to do to help him more effectively. The list included information about himself that he'd never shared with her, such as: "When you talk to me like a child as you give me my pills, it's hard for me to hear you. Instead, if you explain to me how you're reeling from all you have to do, it opens my heart and then I'm responsive to you."

This information was a revelation to Rose. When faced with adversity, her coping style (see chapter 3) made her good at accomplishing such tasks as briskly doling out medications. But she had focused so much on efficiency that she forgot about showing compassion for all Dan was going through. Rose was a "thinker."

Dan went on to write: "I'm a man who responds to touch instead of words. Touch my hand or my face when you tell me what you want me to do. That helps me hear you. I want hugging and cuddling instead of orders. Then I know you care. I don't feel so contrary and understand that of course I have to take my pills."

Another entry in the notebook read: "When I can't sleep at night, I look for you, and I don't always know how to tell you I need you. Please understand I'm struggling because I don't know how to say these things."

Rose was so touched by Dan's words that she began to cry softly. "I had no idea you felt this way," she told him. "I'm so sorry I haven't done better for you. I really love you. I want you well." As for Dan, he was thrilled at her acceptance of his suggestions and her willingness to change.

When I first saw Dan's instruction list, I immediately named it the "Husband Manual." Since then, I've recommended the idea to many couples. You may want to try it yourself. All you have to do is ask your man to write his own Husband (or Partner) Manual, which is literally an instruction guide for taking care of him. You ask him to tell you what he needs—and what you're doing that he would like you to change. You want to know exactly how to talk to him so he can hear you.

We tend to take care of others in the style in which *we* would like to be taken care of, but men often want something totally different. For example, perhaps he tunes you out when you're bossy. Like Dan, he reacts only to your tone, which pushes his emotional buttons. Then he proceeds to put you down or explode. Rose quickly learned that when she was gentle with Dan, she got patience and appreciation in return. The idea is to be authentic, of course, but make sure to give him what he needs, not what you *think* he needs, and only what you realistically are capable of.

To make use of the Husband Manual, you do have to temper your sensitivity to hearing criticism and be willing to make some changes in your own behavior. It may seem unfair and it may be difficult. But remember, when *he* does better, *you* do better.

Encouraging Partnership

Gently try to persuade him to collaborate with you on developing this manual. If he isn't the expressive type, he can treat it the way he would a business meeting and write out an agenda. The goal is to help him become your partner. Then it will be easier to work together in the long run. Chances are, it will not only make life together easier, it will bring you closer.

For example, his manual might include tips on timing. Perhaps he prefers that you tend to his incision first thing in the morning but leave serious discussions until after breakfast, when he's had his coffee and is ready to deal with the day. Maybe he wants you to give him back rubs late in the afternoon to relax him. Dan gave Rose permission to leave him alone. He wrote: "I don't need you all the time. Let me be instead of constantly asking if I'm okay."

The Husband Manual allows your mate to say, "I'm sick and I know you don't know what to do. Here's how I like it." It provides a clear road map to effective caregiving. When you know what to do, you can feel competent instead of scared and overwhelmed.

After Rose read Dan's list, she was able to explain why she acted bitter and angry at times. She was terrified that he would need a catheter after surgery and that she would not be able to handle it properly when he came home. She might make a mistake that could hurt him. Dan immediately suggested, "Why don't we hire a nurse to come in and do it?"

I encouraged him to go even further, saying, "You're still well. Why don't *you* call an agency and arrange for a nurse so that Rose doesn't have to worry about it?"

Rose had to stop bossing Dan and start expressing her feelings more. Dan had to take more responsibility for tasks, take his own pills, call the nurse, and do more of what he could. This change would ease her anxiety.

I pointed out to Rose, "I think you've been doing the best you know how to do. You didn't want to burden Dan by telling him you're scared. As a result, you hid your fear, became impatient, and gave him orders. If you tell him how anxious you are, you will sound much softer." Rose trusted the advice, and Dan beamed. The Husband Manual opened up discussion of important issues for this couple and allowed them to begin to feel empathy for each other.

It is far less lonely to face fears together, and doing so is truly transformational. You're less likely to act out in negative ways as Rose did, and less likely to feel petrified and want to run away.

A Manual for You?

The Husband Manual provides critical information you can use to improve communication with your mate. But it's equally important to give him information about *you* and what you need. You may want to try a Wife Manual, where you can bring up issues such as his constant complaining. You may think, "If he whines again, I'll scream." In a Wife Manual, you might say, "Honey, I know you are miserable, but when you complain all the time, I feel inadequate and unappreciated. Instead, can you tell me exactly what you need?" Complaining is usually a smokescreen for his difficulty in asking for help. If you explain what he has to do to help you, you help him more.

Or your mate may be the silent type. When he doesn't talk to you, it may drive you to distraction. You can say, "It helps me to know what you want. It makes me feel less alone."

KNOCKING DOWN WALLS

AFTER THE ACTOR Christopher Reeve died, his widow, Dana, spoke of their ability to feel deep emotions and discuss them during his long illness. "We had no room for walls," she said during her TV appearance on *The Oprah Winfrey Show*.

The Husband Manual and the Wife Manual are ways to start knocking down walls in your relationship. Another way is to mourn the life you used to have and talk with your mate about what you've both lost. It's difficult to do, requiring communication skills and testing the intimacy between you. A wonderful way to start a discussion is to say, without blaming or complaining, "I miss playing tennis (or gardening or dancing) with you." He may take this opening to mention all that he misses. Who knows? You may have a healing dialogue and even a good cry together. It is then that you can begin to focus on what you *do* have. This process prevents your getting stuck in what was and mired in bitterness, and allows you to move on with life as it is now. It opens the door to problem solving.

Perhaps one of your losses is family celebrations and other events he can't or won't attend. Although you can go by yourself, it isn't the same without him. When he consents to visit friends, he wants to leave after a half hour. You're deprived of the rest of a delightful afternoon. Instead of allowing your irritation to build, why not tell him as calmly as you can after you get home,

"I miss leisurely visits with José and Maria. I miss going to weddings. Let's figure out how to handle the next occasion in a way we both can benefit."

When you speak in these terms and stick to an "I" message (as in, "I miss—"), you remove the sting of criticism, which only makes him defensive. Compare an "I miss" statement with something like, "You never want to go out," which to him may feel like blame. "I miss" takes ownership of your own feelings and may help him feel secure enough to do the same. Maybe he'll admit that he's afraid he won't feel well when he goes out, or that he doesn't feel safe enough when away from home for more than a short time. You learn that he isn't just acting cranky and selfish. He's frightened.

This information sheds a whole new light on what has happened—and may turn your crabby feelings toward him into loving ones. Such interactions help head off or dissipate anger between you and bring you closer together. If you are really centered and savvy, you might even talk about ways to allay his fears, such as agreeing to leave home for only a limited amount of time and keeping a cell phone available for emergencies. You want to do what you realistically can—no more. If he can't tolerate (or isn't capable of) such a conversation, accept that you can only go so far. You may have to talk with someone else you trust instead.

LEARNING TO COLLABORATE

IF YOU VIEW your mate's illness as "his problem," your marriage has a higher risk for distance and even failure. Turning his illness into a transformational experience for both of you requires a collaborative effort. The struggle becomes "ours," and one of the priorities is to become the best-functioning team you can.

Florence and her husband usually work well as a team. They fight at times, but they also regroup later to solve problems. "He's very persistent and creative, good at figuring out little things to do that make a difference in improving his quality of life. I'm in charge of keeping perspective. The glass is often half empty for him, but I focus on the positive things going on—that he's walking better and getting stronger. I think it does help him," she says.

If you find that you and your mate resist collaboration, try to ask yourself why. One husband I know had two heart attacks but always went to the doctor alone. His wife refused to go with him because she didn't want to face how seriously ill he was. When he came home, she'd then get angry with him for failing to ask the doctor the right questions. The real issue—her fear—was never addressed. In therapy she had to learn to talk about it with him, me, or someone else; otherwise she would have remained a backseat driver. Her old behavior denigrated the relationship, because he never got it right. The real problem was her, not him.

TAKING THE FOCUS OFF ILLNESS

THERE IS ALWAYS the danger that your partner's condition will become the sole focus of your relationship and take over your marriage. Try to remain vigilant about boundaries and make sure that doesn't happen. Once he's recovered or the crisis has passed, find other topics to talk about instead of dwelling on dire outcomes. If he has a long-term chronic condition, you can still carve out a piece of your life where illness does not intrude. Bolster other healthy qualities in your relationship. If possible, you can play board games, visit children or friends or have them visit you, listen to music together, and talk with each other.

A good way to keep your relationship alive and growing is to build in a date night as a couple. If your mate is too ill to get out, be creative. Rent a movie, prepare a special dinner, or order in if that's more interesting or less exhausting for you. Spouses or partners often see each other in bathrobes, so it's important to get dressed up and look your best. A change in clothes can help you change your perspective.

Talk about what connects you. If a "date" isn't possible, remembering events and talking about your life together is. Reminisce about your shared experiences to help remind you why you're going through this. Your history together cements your marriage—the places you've lived, the children you've raised, the joys and heartaches. One useful activity is to sit down together with your photograph album. As you flip through the pages, you'll recall memories that nourish your relationship.

If you're in a second or even third marriage or significant relationship, you may have a shorter history together. You can still think of little things the two of you can laugh about, like the romantic roadside picnic when the tablecloth blew away and the car broke down. Remember who you are and why you chose each other. Think about ways you can give to each other.

LOOKING AT A ROLE MODEL

TRANSFORMATIONAL LOVE HAS carried Sam and Nina through many years of his worsening heart disease, severe complications of diabetes, including amputation, and other daunting medical issues. I consider them a model for other couples. His sieges with illness have actually drawn them closer. They've chosen a life of low stress, in which they can spend more time together without losing their livelihoods as freelance artists. They've moved from an urban area to a quiet country town, giving up a lot of what they thought they needed, such as a rich cultural life of theater and concerts. Life's necessities can alter one's priorities.

Sam and Nina have both grown and changed within their relationship. Sam, who tends to be a stoic, has had to learn to let Nina help him rather than take his feelings of helplessness out on her. She tries to curb her tendency to overdo caregiving, and she now understands what it means to him to be able to do as much as possible himself.

Transformational love is not perfect, and Sam and Nina are not a perfect couple. They have struggled and continue to do so. They live with the anxiety of not knowing what comes next. But they share a deep, abiding love that prevails because they are able to do enough things right in their marriage enough of the time. They're both able to feel the joy of having a life together and appreciate their ability to resolve conflicts, solve problems, communicate with respect and humor, and be patient with each other. Nina is a generous person who has altered her life, not given it up.

Their relationship is all the more admirable because they have a long second marriage, with a blended family of four grown children. If they can achieve and maintain their depth of connection with each other, perhaps it is possible for you and your partner, too.

SEVEN WAYS TO GET CLOSER

TRANSFORMATIONAL LOVE INVOLVES humanity (and sometimes humility) in marriage and significant relationships, as well as a confluence of body and mind, heart and soul. It enables you to expand your capacity for unconditional love. Here are some ways to nourish the closeness between you:

1. Communicate, but use judgment.

Communication does not mean making hurtful comments to him about things over which he has no control. If you feel sick of being the sole breadwinner, the maid, and the custodian of the checkbook, maybe you can keep those feelings to yourself or share them with a friend instead of expressing them to your mate. He already feels bad enough about his helplessness. Otherwise, however, try to talk kindly together about the impact of his illness on your life together, and your worries and fears about the future. Such discussions can help you adjust to changes and live a more fulfilling life.

When you master communication skills, you're also less likely to blame him—for being sick, getting older, or betraying you by no longer being the man he was. Blame is a common tool spouses use to avoid facing their true issues. For example, if he's at home and you're working, he may feel you don't spend enough time with him, when the real issue is that he feels unlovable and fears you'll abandon him. You may feel you need breathing space for yourself. Therapy can help you build empathy for each other and find ways both of you can be happy. Perhaps if he has more company when you're gone, he may feel less deprived of your presence. Or you can agree on setting time priorities. Try having lunch or watching a movie together several times a week.

A competent therapist can work magic for both of you. He or she can understand the changes in your life and the conflicts that beset you and your partner. A therapist can also help you express what you feel about what is happening and learn more effective communication skills.

Imagine you're having trouble with your golf swing. Then a coach comes along and says, "Why don't you turn your wrist a little differently?" That small change makes a huge difference. Try to think of a therapist as a wise and objective observer and educator who gives you a different spin on life.

2. Avoid bickering.

There are times where anger is appropriate. But genuine anger is different from bickering, which is a form of nitpicking. Bickering tends to be unproductive and focuses on unimportant details, as opposed to genuine anger about something major, such as a medical mistake. Bickering is often leaked-out resentment, and it can make solving problems next to impossible.

It's the little unaddressed annoyances that often become insurmountable mountains in a relationship. Be aware of irritants between you and your mate, and cut off bickering at the pass. Otherwise it can chip away at the bond between you until there's nothing left.

Kim realized that she dreaded getting up in the morning because bickering began as soon as she had to dispense her husband Charley's medications. He balked at the sheer number of pills he had to take. She understood his frustration, but she also knew he needed the pills to control his condition. Every time she approached him with the meds, he exploded at her. She felt furious with him and argued back. Then they'd avoid each other for hours.

Eventually she thought of a solution: delegate the job to his part-time aide. He wouldn't argue with *her*. That helped, but not entirely. Finally, one morning Kim put her arms around Charley and wouldn't let him go. "We're stuck," she told him. "We have to figure out together how you can take the meds without our fighting about it. Our bickering is killing our relationship. I'll try to be more understanding about what a pain it is to take all of these pills. But I need you to understand how hurt and angry I get when you yell at me. That has to stop." Ten minutes later, he told her, "What you said meant a lot to me."

Although Charley's complaining didn't cease completely, his yelling did. Equally important, his comments didn't bother her as much as they used to. They both felt better and more loving. There's another reason to work on this issue: a study of married couples by scientists at Ohio State University suggests that consistent conflict in the couple relationship hinders a mate's physical healing.

3. Choose the best environment in which to talk.

Pay attention to the times and places of discussion with your partner. If you need to address a difficult issue, such as money troubles, the last place to bring them up is in the bedroom. One room in the house should be a place of safety and refuge.

On the other hand, the bedroom may be perfect for quiet, intimate conversation. One couple has some of their best talks in bed on weekend mornings, when they are both relaxed. "Sometimes he'll start talking out of the blue. If not, I'm able to ask questions in a nonthreatening way and talk about my own concerns, which leads him to open up. Afterward, we always feel closer and happier."

During a weekend away at an inn, after he had recuperated from surgery, they were talking in bed at seven a.m. about the room décor and how nice it was to have a couch near the window. "You know, I had trepidation about coming here," he suddenly confided. "About what," she asked. "Was it driving a distance for the first time?" And his answer was yes. It took that calm environment for him to feel safe enough to admit his anxiety. You and your mate may also find a different time or place that fosters intimacy. Take advantage of it.

4. Know how he operates.

This is the time to better understand your partner's needs and motivations, both conscious and unconscious. He is and always will remain a different person from you. That's part of why you married him. For example, you may grieve losses by reaching out for support, while he may turn inward for strength or outward to God. Every couple struggles with such differences. This is an ideal time for a brief period in couples therapy. Why struggle when you both have enough to deal with? Let a professional help you find ways to work together. When he's ill and he changes, you're forced to change, too. Intimacy flourishes when the two of you make conscious choices together.

5. **Change activity patterns.**

Try anything that breaks your routine and helps you and your partner find a new way to relate and connect. You have to be innovative and make adjustments, but your life doesn't have to stop. If you can, get away. Perhaps friends have a weekend house or city apartment you can use for a few days. When it's possible to travel, take a trip together.

I think of Pam and her husband, who was in a wheelchair after an accident. The calamity didn't diminish his zest for life—or hers. When told he needed surgery, they scheduled a cruise to the Greek Islands for after his recovery. The planning distracted them from fears about the operation and also gave them something to look forward to. Yes, they once took adventure vacations in Africa, and they can't do that anymore. Yet within limits, they live the best life they can.

Not every man is as open to travel ideas as Pam's husband. Another husband balked at his wife's plans for a vacation six weeks after his cancer surgery. Even though his doctors supported the plan, he offered other excuses. He was afraid he wouldn't be well enough to go. His wife took charge and finally persuaded him to change his mind with the argument: "*I* need this trip. Do it for me.

We'll take out travel insurance as a hedge in case we have to cancel."

Not only did they take the vacation, he now praises her for ignoring his objections and doing what she thought was best. The trip was healing and rejuvenating for both of them.

Beware of falling into the trap of thinking, "We can't go anywhere." You may have many options you've never considered. For example, the Internet offers travel sites for people with disabilities.

Take care not to isolate yourselves as a couple, either. A shared activity with social benefits can be ideal. Some couples become active in the organization specific to his disease and enlarge their social circle at the same time. These groups can be especially useful if you're a younger couple who, because of what you've been through, feels different and out of sync with others your age, and wise beyond your years. Or you can both get involved in politics, community activities, or your place of worship, where you meet new people together. Such shared involvements can give your relationship a stimulating boost.

6. Pay attention to your wounds.

We all carry hurts from childhood that affect how we give or receive love as adults. When illness strikes and the balance of your relationship shifts, old fears can reemerge. Under stress we all regress. You may have had a childhood fear of being abandoned, which causes you to want to run from your partner before he dies and leaves you first. Or because you grew up feeling emotionally smothered or controlled, you may try to spend every second with your partner or overdo caregiving. Your partner may respond to the same fears in his own way, by demanding your constant attention.

These reactions are normal, but avoid getting stuck in them. If you feel yourself pulling away from your partner, watch out. He needs you more than ever. If necessary, take a break and get some distance for yourself, or seek support to help you hang in there.

7. **Keep a sense of humor.**

In his best-selling book, *Anatomy of an Illness as Perceived by the Patient,* Norman Cousins wrote about combating life-threatening illness through humor and patient participation. Research confirms that laughter can be therapeutic. Dr. Lee Berk and Dr. Stanley Tan at Loma Linda University in California have studied the effects of laughter on the immune system and found that laughter boosts immune function and reduces blood pressure and stress hormones. The endorphins released when we laugh also make us feel better.

I believe in the healing power of laughter. I've told couples, "Crying together touches your soul. Laughing together brings you grace."

REACHING THE OBJECTIVE

WHEN YOU WORK together and move toward mutual help, you increase the chances of turning your mate's illness into a transformational experience for both of you. A deeper spiritual health and connection can take place. Some of the time you may become his coach, cheering him on or setting limits. Try to achieve the most loving, productive collaboration you possibly can. Your relationship can be either a significant source of stress or one of support. Make sure it's the latter.

Reflections

- *Do your best to build intimacy between you and your partner.*

- *Be your authentic self.*

- *Remember, the better he does emotionally, the better it is for you.*

- *Give your mate what he needs, not just what you think he needs.*

- *Communicate constructively, and clarify what you expect from each other.*

12

Your Sex Life
and Serious Illness

Is there sex after prostate cancer, heart attack, stroke, or other illnesses? This is often a troubling question for couples facing a serious diagnosis or already living with limitations. How could it not be? Lovemaking tends to be a delicate issue for most couples, even when they are healthy. When your partner is ill, physiological changes in him and psychological shifts in both of you add an extra challenge.

The impact of his illness on lovemaking depends on a number of factors, including the nature and stage of his condition, type of treatment, and perhaps most important, your sex life *before* he got sick. Sexual issues that existed earlier are likely to be magnified. In most cases, these complications needn't destroy your sex life if it is important to your relationship. Although adjustments may have to be made, sexual connection can be maintained.

ILLNESS AND YOUR PARTNER'S
SEXUAL FUNCTIONING

LET'S BE REALISTIC. A major blow to your mate's health changes your situation as a couple and has ramifications for the quality of your sex life. Making love involves a delicate balance among senses, heart, and mind. It's difficult enough to relax and feel desire when things are normal, let alone when both of you are buffeted by the worry and stress that accompany illness. The medical condition itself may also interfere with lovemaking. For example, prostate complexities, diabetes, high blood pressure, arteriosclerosis (hardening of the arteries), chronic liver problems, or kidney disease and dialysis may cause erectile dysfunction. Pain and hormonal issues may affect his performance and interest in sex.

Then he must contend with emotional and psychological issues. Imagine what a heart attack does to a man's confidence. He may fear that exertion of any kind will kill him. Twenty-five percent of male heart attack patients give up sex entirely, and another 50 percent have sex less frequently than they did before the attack. In 80 percent of such cases, these changes in lifestyle are unnecessary, writes Saul H. Rosenthal, MD, author of *The New Sex Over 40*.

Depression after any illness dampens a man's ardor, as can anxiety and loss of self-esteem. Treatment side effects may be another complication. Cancer therapy may lower sexual desire and can cause erectile problems or inability to achieve orgasm. Drugs such as antihypertensives, antidepressants, and ulcer medications can also affect function. The more you know about what's causing problems and the options available, the more likely you are to preserve your sex life.

YOUR OWN ISSUES

YOU FACE SEXUAL challenges at the same time your partner does. The anxiety and exhaustion that go hand in hand with caregiving are not exactly aphrodisiacs. It may be difficult to feel sexy if you're concerned about touching his surgical incision or some other tender area, or causing an attack of some kind while making love. No wonder it's common for desire to decline (or disappear) when taking care of an ill mate. Yet sex begins in the brain. The right frame of mind is a powerful asset.

Sex is life affirming. My client Mark, age sixty, had to undergo several complicated surgeries, and every time he came home from the hospital, he wanted sex. For him, this was a statement that he was very much alive. The mechanics of intercourse weren't easy for Mark. His wife didn't particularly feel like a femme fatale at this time, yet she eagerly joined in lovemaking. To her it meant he was truly on the road to recovery. "It wasn't the finest sex I ever had, because I worried about hurting his healing wound. But it was memorable nevertheless in its way, because I felt thrilled that he wanted sex. It was an affirmation that we still had a life. We giggled a lot about it afterward," she says.

Effects of Illness on Physical Attraction

A poignant essay by Jennifer Glaser in the *New York Times* detailed how she and her boyfriend found joy in sexual connection as he waged a losing battle with leukemia and endured debilitating treatment. Their active sex life expressed their love and kept them close. "During his lengthy and wholly unsexy illness, he had never ceased to be sexy to me," wrote Glaser. This experience reaches back to the power of transformational love and the ability to embrace what is meaningful and essential.

For another woman, Asha, sexual desire has always been connected more to her husband's sharp mind than to his body. "I've always been attracted to him, but not as a 'hunk' physically. He never looked great at the beach. For me, his magnetism is his personality and intelligence, and his dear face. He is a package." She is able to view him as a whole person, which is a key to preserving attraction.

Not everyone can move through a partner's serious illness as seamlessly. If his condition or treatment causes significant body changes, you may find it difficult to feel physically attracted to him. This is a common and normal reaction. Many women in your position feel the same way. However, your negative feelings can change to positive, loving ones if you are willing to be patient and make some adjustments in your expectations.

Consider Helen, a client of mine who deeply loved her strong, strapping husband, Jerry. When cancer treatment left him looking emaciated, Jerry's body turned her off. After they made love, her feelings of distaste left her filled with self-loathing. Sometimes she left the bedroom in tears. She had always felt protected by his size. Now it seemed she was with a stranger, someone fragile in an unfamiliar body, who could never protect her again.

Fortunately, this couple sought help and eventually were able to resume their sex life. Guilt-ridden about her feelings, Helen entered therapy first and was able to talk about her new sense of vulnerability. After several months in therapy, Helen began to adjust to her husband's new image and even the feel of his body. Gradually she realized that the man she loved, the person he was, was still present; it was only his body that had changed. She started to reshape her expectations and asked Jerry to join us in our sessions. Although Helen couldn't have the robust sex she was accustomed to, she could enjoy a gentler, more sensual version. She discovered new sexual positions that allowed her to achieve satisfaction without any danger of hurting him. For example, previously she preferred the missionary position where she felt protected by her husband's bulk. Instead, she nestled into positions where they faced each other or she gently straddled him. Jerry was able to become more verbally expressive during sex, which excited Helen—and in turn stirred him.

Helen came to realize that Jerry was still the man who brought her breakfast in bed, caressed her hair, and loved her for who she was. He was still a nurturing father to their teenage daughters. These changes, and the evolution of Helen's feelings, took time. I've often thought of this couple's courage and determination. They truly loved each other and worked hard to change their attitudes. They refused to let illness interfere with the physical expression of that love.

WHEN INTERCOURSE IS IMPOSSIBLE

IF YOU'RE FACED with a mate's back surgery, abstinence for a time may be just what the doctor ordered. In fact, you may be so busy with all you have to do and so tired at the end of the day that neither of you is very interested in more than a good-night kiss.

On the other hand, if your mate's illness causes permanent damage or progressive deterioration, lovemaking as you knew it might never be the same again. Yet some couples are endlessly resourceful at finding ways to keep intimacy alive. Sexual intercourse is out of the question for Rita and her husband, a retired Philadelphia fireman, who suffers from chronic obstructive pulmonary disease (COPD). Their very active sex life had to stop, which is a big loss for both of them. Although it isn't easy, they've found many ways to express intimacy. "We aren't dead yet," says Rita. "We play a lot. Sometimes I lift up my shirt and act sexy, and he enjoys it. We can still touch. We hold hands and hug and kiss."

Lovemaking can provide pleasure, comfort, and intimacy, no matter what condition your mate is in. Although they miss intercourse, some couples remember that making love is a process, not just an end goal.

A Florida woman whose artist partner had surgery and other treatments for prostate cancer told me:

Sex is very important to us, and we're still very active in some ways. It's not what it used to be, but it's enough to make us happy. Intercourse is not an option anymore, but he can still have orgasms. We do what we have to do to make ourselves content. I know couples that don't even sleep together. They have separate rooms or beds, but I think they miss a lot. In our case, it's only our bodies that change as we age. Our desires and minds do not.

We laugh and tease each other a lot about things we used to do and can't do anymore. So what? The other night he said, "Come lie in my arms. We haven't done this in a while and I miss it." There are little ways to show affection if you can't do the big ones. The important thing is to know you are still there for each other.

This couple's ability to joke about what they can no longer have is a sign of the strength of their relationship. Unless it is talked about, a no-sex marriage rarely bodes well for the relationship.

If intercourse isn't possible, it's sad that a precious part of your relationship is missing. So it's important to try to face your loss and grieve. Acknowledge it, talk about missing it, and maybe even cry together. Then you can look for creative ways to compensate for what's missing.

People want physical relief, and some partners masturbate in front of each other to make it a shared experience. One wife creeps behind her husband's wheelchair to give him surprise hugs. An eighty-four-year-old woman I know gently pinches her husband's butt when she walks by. Even though he is the more reserved of the two, he now does the same for her. Sex has become sensuality and connectedness instead of a simple thrust.

MAKING DECISIONS

IF YOUR SEX life is one of the major losses of your partner's illness, you have decisions to make. Not everyone cares about sex or wants to stay sexually active. Some women welcome the end of lovemaking, especially if menopause has affected their desire and changed their sexual response.

Many others wish to remain as sexual as possible. When help is available for your mate, you may want him to seek it—although he may balk at the idea. Many men deny their sexual problems or are embarrassed to talk to a physician about them. You may have to read between the lines to understand your partner's resistance and develop a strategy to change his mind.

I remember working with one husband who refused to use Viagra. As a result, their sex life died. In the course of therapy he confided a secret to me that he'd kept from his wife. He had already tried Viagra—once. But he experienced a vision disturbance, a blue haze, which can be a side effect of the drug, caused by constriction of blood vessels. This man saw little blue dots, which scared him mightily. I couldn't blame him for refusing to take Viagra again, and I was able to say, "You can try another product that doesn't have that effect."

I suggested several other similar drugs on the market. Although he tried a few and they worked, he never felt comfortable using medication. Eventually, both he and his wife decided to return to making love without drugs. They became accustomed to his less erect penis. With an attitude shift, they found both of them could live with satisfaction that was "good enough."

In fact, the attitude toward prescription medications for erectile dysfunction has changed. Some men find they don't work as well as advertised—and there can be troublesome side effects. In such cases, perhaps nonmedical sex aids can be helpful. If sex was good before illness, some adult videos and toys can be assets.

Some men visit adult Web sites when they feel sexually inadequate during or after illness. These sites can be useful for adding spice to your love life. But the risk is addiction, which can interfere with, rather than enhance, your sexual relationship. If such a problem develops, it's important to seek help.

Do You Want to Maintain Your Sexuality?

A significant number of adult women masturbate and some women I've talked to do turn to their vibrators as a useful friend. One of them puts it this way: "It's important to me to stay sexual and have orgasms. I don't know what the future will bring."

Brita, whose sex life disappeared after her husband had a stroke, told me, "It was a combination of the stroke itself and all the medications. That's a hard thing, but what are you going to do? I don't have an answer. We always had a good sex life, and I miss it. I do masturbate. At least it keeps me sexually alive."

Another woman believes that masturbation protects her from having an affair. "This way I can live with the loss of our sex life," she says. "Without it, I'd feel too deprived. I'm happy I don't have hang-ups about this."

Some women reject masturbation for religious or other reasons. They may have been taught that sexual pleasure is acceptable only when pursuing procreation. One wife abstains for reasons of control. "It's better this way," she explains. "If I masturbated, I'm afraid I wouldn't be able to contain my feelings." Only you can decide what's right for you.

COMMUNICATING WITH YOUR MATE

DESPITE THE BARRAGE of explicit material all around us, many couples have a terrible time talking with each other about sexual concerns. When your mate is sick, it can feel doubly uncomfortable to raise the subject. Although you don't want to deliberately hurt his feelings, you may distress him by discussing this sensitive subject. The answer is to speak lovingly, honestly, and thoughtfully about what's really happening between you. It can feel like a risk to do so, but it's a risk worth taking to keep love alive.

Bring up sex concerns when you're both dressed and outside the bedroom. Here are some common issues that can arise during and after illness and how to handle them:

- **Issue:** He might benefit from erectile enhancers but won't try them.

  He may remember himself as a young stud or as he was before he got sick, and might consider sex aids for "wimps." Bartering is a creative way to get through to him. Tell him, "I'd really like you to try one of these products. What would you like me to do in return?" Offer to make his favorite dish or watch the football game with him on TV in exchange. If he's afraid of side effects, which can be a legitimate fear, suggest he try half a dose.

  Some men object because it feels like too much of a commitment to fill a prescription and get a supply of pills. If you suspect that's what's going on, you can suggest he ask the doctor for a sample. Tell him, "Then you can try a few different drugs and we can see which works best." A sample seems more like an experiment, and it's a good way to ease into the idea. Assure him you love him, no matter what, and point out that many men try such treatments.

- **Issue:** He refuses to consider a penile implant or other options if erectile enhancers can't help him.

  If this is important to you, try to sweet-talk your partner and explain how much you want to be with him physically. A little seduction can help. You may also have to do some research to show him the different options that are available and discuss the pros and cons.

If he still refuses to try products or devices that can help him, you may feel abandoned and grow furious at what you feel is a stubborn partner. Anger only beats down his self-esteem and is not your best course of action. Instead, try to stay calm and understand what he's going through. In the end, it's his decision. Like the couple in the blue haze story, there are cases where simple relaxation and a change in attitude may be the best medicine of all.

Of course, sometimes he wants the implant but *you're* frightened for his health. You may worry that he can't withstand another medical procedure. In a case like this, one partner can carry the courage as the other holds the fear.

■ **Issue:** He tries to become a sexual athlete.

Some men want to prove that nothing has changed, that there is no difference in their performance. Their gymnastics can scare you. At such times it's useful to tell your partner he satisfies you just the way he is. He doesn't have to be a contortionist or jump through hoops.

■ **Issue:** He's frightened after surgery and makes you nervous.

Your mate may be afraid to initiate sex or have trouble getting erections because of anxiety. As a result, you worry he'll have an attack. Go slowly here. Realize that there's no time clock, no scorekeeper, no judge. It can be hard for him to regain his confidence, and the process can't be rushed.

In an opposite reaction, sometimes a man feels so happy to be alive and able to perform sexually that he wants to go out and have affairs. This is devastating news to his partner. Some women may consider giving permission "in view of all he's been through."

There's a difference, however, between fantasy and action. If he tells you, "Now that I'm okay, I wish I could go out and sleep with other women," realize that infidelity can have huge consequences for both of you individually and as a couple. This is a case where a therapist or a member of the clergy can help you explore the ramifications.

Unexpected Fallout

More frequently, when intercourse isn't possible, your man may feel compelled to give *you* permission to have an affair. Such an offer stunned Linda, a woman in her late forties. After her husband was paralyzed in a boating accident, he told her, "You're still a young woman. If at any time you want a lover—go ahead and do it. I understand. I just don't want to know about it."

Linda's reaction was shock and anger. "I told him, 'If you think I married you because of your penis, you're so wrong. Thanks for the offer, but no thanks.'" She misses their sex life. She masturbates and uses a vibrator, and sometimes fantasizes, "What if—?" But for her, infidelity is not an option.

Another wife has never discussed the issue of an affair with her husband yet is certain he would approve if she wanted one. "I just couldn't do it," she says. Even though she is bitter about the burden of caregiving, she believes an affair would be a betrayal she could not live with.

Conversely, some people find sexual fulfillment and even love for themselves outside of their marriage and still remain good caregivers. This is a matter of personal morality, conscience, and religious belief.

SEVEN WAYS TO DEAL WITH
SEXUAL CHALLENGES

SEX IS PART of the fabric of life and can actually be therapeutic unless ruled out for medical reasons. Most couples find that sex revitalizes their bond and refuels them emotionally. Here's how to maximize your sexual connection if you want that, or adjust if you don't:

1. **Find out the facts.**

   It's all too easy to believe unfounded rumors and misinformation about sexual functioning after illness or treatment. Avoid this trap and talk with your doctor or other health professionals. Get over any feelings of embarrassment about raising this important but often touchy subject. Sometimes the doctor is embarrassed, too. When you talk about your sex life, you give him or her permission to weigh in.

   Try not to hold back; ask all the questions on your mind. If your mate needs surgery for prostate cancer, can his nerves be spared to prevent impotence? If he can't perform, is it because of a medicine he's taking? Can he switch to a different antihypertensive or antidepressant if his present drug affects sexual function? Can drugs for erectile dysfunction help? Are there other possibilities?

2. **Don't make assumptions.**

   Although some sexual issues apply regardless of the illness, others vary with the diagnosis. Educate yourself about what is and isn't possible in your mate's specific case. He (and you) may be needlessly fearful that sexual activity can harm him or isn't an option. Learn what to expect. For example, many people who undergo heart surgery experience a period of depression afterward. If you don't know about this possibility, you may experience his lack of desire as a hurtful rejection.

Web sites for organizations such as the American Heart Association, Alzheimer's Association, American Cancer Society, and National Kidney Foundation offer online information on relevant sexual issues. They may also have social workers available to talk with you about the subject. This help can be especially useful if your mate exhibits changes in sexual behavior that are actually symptoms of the disease.

For example, one husband had a stroke that left him physically potent but affected him mentally. His behavior and attitude changed. "We never stopped making love," his wife reported, "but his needs and mine were different. He had always been a very giving lover in the past, but for a long time he lost interest in satisfying me. That's finally changed."

Brain changes may cause loss of inhibition, and some Alzheimer's patients may expose themselves, masturbate in public, or become sexually aggressive toward a partner. This can be very painful for you. The man you married is there in body but not in mind.

A support group specific to the disease can be helpful for such situations, and for dealing with your feelings if you are no longer attracted to him. Some of the best people to talk with are those who have been there before.

3. **Change your thinking about what sex is all about.**

As sexuality wanes, sensuality gains. There are lots of ways to have sex besides intercourse. If the mechanics of making love become difficult and he can't get an erection (even with medication), your methods and techniques for loving may need to change. Try to be innovative. Perhaps your fingers can do the walking and talking. Oral sex and even sex toys may be what you choose. For many people this is unfamiliar ground, but it is an opportunity to keep your affection alive.

One option you may wish to explore is Tantric sex. This involves the Eastern idea that the ultimate goal in sex is not intercourse but rather how long you can sustain intimacy without ejaculation or orgasm. Regardless of the state of his physical body, the two of you can connect.

4. Protect the attraction between you.

There is a unique magnetic relationship between two people who are in love with each other. Mystery is part of the attraction. Romantic attachment is a fragile bond that can't always stand up to his problems, yours, and the indignities of patient care. The experience can desexualize the image of who your partner is and his role in your life.

That's a reason to encourage his own self-care whenever possible. If that's not possible, try to put limits on tasks you perform for him, and have someone else tend to his bodily needs. This may be necessary to protect your relationship as a couple.

Long-term caregiving duties can smother sexual interest and even change the couple relationship to more of a parent-child connection than that of a husband and wife. This was the case with Moira. She was repelled by what should have been a relatively simple task—helping her mate, a school principal, put on support hose when his legs swelled.

"There was something about the touch of his body when putting on the compression stockings that killed my personal attraction to him," she recalls. "It also didn't help that I had to bring the urinal all the time. Sometimes it spilled, and he was sticky. Now there's no sex at all. It just died. He wants to kiss me sometimes, but I don't want to do that anymore. I live with companionship only."

Try not to let this happen to you. Instead, push against feelings of shyness or prudishness, and seek professional help in adjusting to the new situation, before your intimate relationship is contaminated beyond recall.

5. Claim your sexuality.

If you think about and want sex when your husband is seriously ill, you aren't selfish, uncaring, or a bad person, no matter what those voices in your head may tell you. You're normal. (He may even want sex, too, but it may not be possible at this time.) And you both may be having an active fantasy life. What if you considered sharing your fantasies? Perhaps doing so would help the two of you to have fun and communicate in new ways.

Sometimes you will have to alter your expectations. But can you find ways to still feel desirable? He may not be able to engage in intercourse, but that doesn't mean he isn't aware of you as a woman. One wife buys pretty lingerie because it makes her feel good, and her husband appreciates it even though coitus is not possible. He still lets her know she's desirable. She told me, "Just the other day I walked by, and he said, 'You've still got the best pair of legs in town.' That feels good when you're fifty-eight."

6. Fight for your sex life if it's important to you.

The obstacles to having satisfying sex may sometimes seem overwhelming, but you aren't as helpless as you may feel. You may have to be proactive if your partner fears rejection because he doesn't perform the way he used to and may not satisfy you. He may need reassurance that you want him. But be sensitive. There's a fine line between encouragement and pressure on him to perform.

If vaginal dryness is a problem for you, you may want to talk with your doctor about the newest and safest use of hormones. Lubricants, moisturizers, and other products can help as well. Today, exotic massage oils, edible body paints, and other sex enhancers are becoming available at the corner drugstore and at chain stores. And don't forget to talk with other women, who can be great sources of information on options.

Make it easier on both of you. Turn off the TV. Routinely watching your favorite shows in the bedroom can diminish your sex life. It becomes too easy to stare at the screen instead of turning to each other. Pay attention to your environment, and make it as sensual as possible. Dim the lights, wear provocative lingerie, light candles, and draw a bath. Popular women's magazines blare this information because it does help.

Smart timing works, too. Make love when you are fresh, not tired. For many couples that means the morning, but we all have our own optimum times. If pain is an issue for your mate, the American Academy of Family Physicians recommends that he take pain medication a half hour before having sex. Wait two hours after a meal to make love. Excessive alcohol and cigarette smoking should be avoided, as both can cause sexual difficulties.

7. Be true to yourself and him.

For some, sex has never been pleasurable—or not pleasurable enough to become a priority. If that describes you and your mate, you may be quite willing to accept the end of your sex life. That's your decision. However, it remains important to maintain affection between you. All human beings have a need for touch and intimacy. If that need goes unmet, both of you might end up feeling physically and emotionally isolated. Regularly assure your partner that you love him. One wife tells her mate over and over again, "You're the only man for me." Whatever words you choose, remember, he needs to hear them.

WHAT MATTERS

IF YOUR MATE'S illness occurs in midlife or beyond, you may have dealt with the changes and frustrations of your own menopause or his prostate problems. The advent of his cancer, heart disease, or other serious conditions may compound the challenges.

Yet sex in any form helps you stay connected to each other. Expect adjustment issues in the bedroom. Realize that everyone in your situation has them and that there are many ways to love him. Can you be happy enough with the sex you have?

Reflections

- *Misunderstandings and misinformation can needlessly limit your sex life. Get the facts.*

- *You and your partner may have to alter your sexual expectations, but satisfying surprises may be in store, too.*

- *Make love, not only intercourse. Meaningful sex is more than performance.*

- *Accept your feelings, whatever they are, but get help early if negative feelings are driving you away from your mate.*

- *Use what works for you as a couple. Only the two of you can determine what that is.*

PART FOUR

Taking Care of You

13

Coping with Your Emotions

It's hard to stay steady when you and your partner are sailing through turbulent waters. Under stress, you just can't fit society's glorified image of you as a saint. You may experience an array of difficult emotions and sometimes behave in unfamiliar ways. The question becomes: How can you handle distressing feelings and stop them from interfering with what is required of you?

During your partner's illness, there are productive and unproductive ways to cope. Here are some common emotions that are likely to challenge you and ways you can handle them.

ANXIETY AND FEAR

WHEN LIFE GRABS you by the throat, fear and anxiety are sure to follow. Fear is a painful feeling of impending danger: "I'm afraid he'll have another heart attack (or his cancer will recur)." In contrast, anxiety is often a vague state of apprehension, an unfocused nervousness or constant worry; something you can't quite name is bothering you. Both feelings can seem inter- changeable in the turmoil of your mate's illness. And make no mistake—you are going to experience them. Just about everyone in your situation does. Your mate is your other half, your pri- mary support. If you have a good marriage, your emotional safety net crashes when he's ill. Even if your relationship isn't made in heaven, your confidence and equilibrium are still likely to be lost, replaced by a pervasive awareness of what happened (or could happen) in your world.

Anxiety at this time usually stems from fear that he'll be dis- abled, that you'll be left alone, that this ordeal will never end, or other related terrors. Although anxiety may be unavoidable in the moment, it can be contained. Some reactions to anxiety can stand in your way, such as:

The "What-if" Syndrome

Many people, no matter how smart and capable they may be, obsess over what *might* occur—which stops them from acting effectively. This happened to one of my clients after her mate developed a respiratory infection that spiraled out of control. When told he faced complex treatment and a long hospital stay, she visualized astronomical bills that would wipe out their sav- ings, despite Medicare coverage. She agonized for two weeks over impending financial ruin, until one day she finally confided in her son. "I'm afraid Medicare covers only a certain amount of time in the hospital, and we have to pay for the rest," she told him. "The bill could be enormous." Her son replied, "You really don't know the facts. Look up the details of coverage on the Internet, or call Medicare and find out."

Afraid of what she might find, she failed to follow this excel- lent advice. Instead, she continued to obsess, until one night she came across a Medicare information guide she had placed on a bookshelf months before. She took a deep breath and checked the hospitalization section. To her relief, Medicare would cover his stay. "I spent weeks with a stiff neck and knotted stomach, worrying for nothing. Why didn't I ask my son for help? What a waste," she told me.

It was indeed a waste of time, energy, and sleep, yet so understandable. Even though this wife functioned successfully in the business world and ordinarily was a first-rate problemsolver, she was debilitated by fear of finding out the facts. Her internal dialogue proceeded along the lines of "What if it's really true?" "What if it's even worse than I think?" When the "what-if" syndrome overtakes you, it slows you down or even stops you in your tracks. It's useful at such times to confront the anxiety or fear and give it a name. Say it out loud: "I'm afraid of—." Although my client didn't realize it at the time, that's what she did when she confided in her son. After their conversation, she eventually did get the facts. If you have trouble speaking the words, try writing them down.

Naming Your Anxiety Works

This is the same technique that helps you deal with your losses. (See chapter 10.) In this case, as you put your worst fear or anxiety into words, you fully experience its impact. This deflates its power and frees you to deal with what you dread. The scenario played out this way for Jennifer, fifty-two, who was haunted by her husband's worsening kidney disease. Because he was not a candidate for a transplant, he faced ever-increasing disability down the road. Frozen in terror, Jennifer didn't know how to help him. She found herself having nightmares about frantically searching for him, and she often cried in her sleep.

Like many people, Jennifer was more afraid to feel the fear that her husband would die than she was of the death itself. We therapists call this "pseudo fear." Jennifer bottled her concerns inside. I helped her understand that she instead had to clearly voice the words "I'm terrified he'll die and leave me." As she looked her fear in the eye, she found it easier to connect with her husband's needs and her own. Her nightmares stopped. She started to sleep.

Denial

This is another common response to fear. When reality is enormously frightening, you may refuse to accept it. You may insist, "This isn't happening," or fantasize, "Somehow this is going to work out." If your mate has a progressive disease, you may deny it's going to get worse. In extreme cases, you can even convince yourself that the tests are wrong or that the doctors don't know what they are talking about.

Imagine learning that your husband, a renowned economist, has been diagnosed with dementia. For Alice, the response was, "That's impossible. He's a genius. Nobody that brilliant could have dementia." Insisting that her husband was just being cantankerous, she told the doctor forthrightly, "You're wrong."

A certain amount of denial can be protective and get you through initially, especially if it propels you into action or keeps your attitude positive. But denial becomes destructive when it stops you from taking important next steps, such as learning all you can about his disease, or investigating supplies and equipment that could improve his quality of life. When denial lingers, trusted family members and friends may start telling you, "Face reality." That's a clue that you need to listen to what they're saying.

After being assaulted with frightening medical information, sometimes people go into shock, which is a form of denial. Imagine that your mate has surgery for a hernia. The doctor walks out of the operating room and tells you, "It's cancer." You may feel so scared that you become numb and can't think. Under this kind of stress your body freezes, your blood pressure may drop, and you feel like an ice cube. Or you may respond like a deer in the headlights, paralyzed and unable to move. The world swirls around you and you're a part of it, but nothing makes sense.

Shock immobilizes you, but there is also a positive aspect. Shock can wrap you in a protective cocoon that allows you to slowly adjust to the new situation. It's the body's way of helping you survive a tough time.

Panic

Senseless emotional frenzy is another response when fear leaks out. Panic overwhelms you and makes you feel impotent, incompetent, or out of control. Some people have tantrums and act like two-year-olds.

Panic may cause your heart to pound, constrict your throat, or stab you in the gut. In severe cases, you may even think you're going to have a coronary or go crazy. Rarely do these fears come true. Or you may wind up lashing out at people who don't deserve your wrath—friends, your kids, or medical staff. If panic stops you from behaving constructively, try some self-talk.

When you feel the pangs stirring, say to yourself, "Whoa, that panicky feeling is here again. Slow down." Because fear constricts breathing, it's also useful to take a deep breath. A sense of humor helps, too. When you're in the midst of a panic attack, laughter requires courage, but it is therapeutic.

This is also a good time to see a therapist or ask your doctor about temporary medication, such as an antidepressant or antianxiety drug.

Hovering

Sometimes the way you cope with anxiety can interfere with your mate's progress in addition to testing your own mental health. If he's seriously ill, it's only human to watch his every move out of fear he'll stumble and fall, forget his meds, or suffer an attack of some kind. As well meaning as your behavior may be, it can undermine his becoming as independent as possible. I recall one husband who was recovering from a quadruple heart bypass. His wife felt so anxious about his condition, she sat at the window every time he went out for a walk. She would watch and wait, afraid he might collapse in the street and not come back.

It was only after the cardiologist warned, "You can't keep looking over his shoulder," that she was able to let go. Instead of wasting her time worrying and waiting, she learned to spend it in a more productive way—nurturing herself. Sometimes she washed her hair or tried new makeup while he was gone. As he was able to go out for longer periods, she visited with a friend or took her grandkids to the movies.

ANGER

YOU'RE PROBABLY GOING to feel anger at times, especially if you're involved in intensive long-term caregiving. "Anger is universal for both partners living with chronic disorders," writes John S. Rolland, MD, in his book *Families, Illness, & Disability*. A key to handling anger is to acknowledge it. That can be very hard to do when you feel pressure to be eternally patient and loving, despite the demands on you. These unrealistic expectations can lead you to hide your anger and cause a great deal of damage to yourself and others.

Your anger may take many directions:

■ *At the condition.* After all, the disease or injury may erode your quality of life and threaten or debilitate the man you love. Alice, the wife who denied that her husband had dementia, actually expressed her rage in a physical way. "The doctor told me to read a book on coping with Alzheimer's disease. When he gave it to me, I felt so angry I threw it across the room," she recalls.

- *At the doctor.* Why didn't the physician save your husband's leg or prevent a recurrence of cancer? One couple did a great deal of research to find the best surgeon in their area to do nerve-sparing surgery for his prostate cancer. Because of the location of the cancer, the nerves couldn't be spared after all. Although warned initially that this could happen, the couple didn't absorb the caveat. Words were no match for the power of denial, and the wife raged at the surgeon nevertheless. It's healthy denial to put such possibilities out of your mind before the operation, but sometimes the worst happens. It's human to rage when it does.

- *At your mate.* It's hard not to blame your mate when he won't exercise as the doctor has ordered, or if he continues to smoke or behaves self destructively in other ways. Of course you want to say to him, "If you'd only lost weight, you wouldn't have had a heart attack." You have a right to express your resentment, but not to a very sick person. You won't like yourself in the morning. People often say, "Why do I feel so mean?" The answer is because you're human.

    You may also feel furious at the way he treats you. If you're knocking yourself out for him, it isn't easy to tolerate his criticism and lack of appreciation for all you do. Be aware, however, that his anger may not be willful. It can be a symptom of his disease. Some conditions, such as stroke, can affect his ability to control emotions.

- *At children, relatives, and friends.* If the people you count on for support aren't around much (or at all), of course you're going to feel angry and abandoned. Or they may criticize you for not doing enough, for making unwise decisions (in their opinion), or for being cold and selfish when you pay attention to your own needs. No one else lives in your shoes. If you feel you're being judged, you have a right to feel mad.

- *At the burden of responsibilities—and what you've given up.* It's one thing if you're involved in endless tasks for a week or a month or two or three. You know it's temporary and that life will eventually return to a semblance of normality. It's something else if your partner becomes disabled permanently and requires ongoing care. That's a heavy load on your shoulders.

Try to give yourself permission to feel and understand your anger in order to get through this difficult period. Transformational love becomes more difficult to achieve unless you can do so. For example, Marina feels angry at the losses in her life since her husband had a stroke at age fifty-five. He can barely walk and can't talk, although his cognitive abilities remain intact. Their life has constricted to the point where they are mostly housebound, except for trips to doctors' appointments and physical therapy. Marina's anger is appropriate, but letting it make her bitter is not.

In order to stay connected with her husband and keep her marriage alive, it would help Marina to talk about her feelings and accept them. She needs to finish mourning the life she used to have by voicing her sadness and all that she misses and finding ways to move on. Her mate can't participate in a discussion, but that's what friends and therapists are for.

Women are often told it "isn't nice" to talk about anger, especially if that wrath is directed toward a sick mate. But you do have to take the lid off to prevent unhealthy consequences. You may not realize that unexpressed anger often leads to a sense of hopelessness that can become depression or evolve into long-term resentment.

Hidden anger often leaks out in other ways, too. We are all familiar with red-in-the-face, screaming-out-loud rage. But some people insist they're fine even as they speak through clenched teeth. Others sigh frequently as if carrying a heavy burden (which of course they are). Or they turn their anger into a kind of martyrdom. It is neither healthy nor effective to behave like a suffering, sacrificial victim.

DEPRESSION: HOPELESSNESS AND HELPLESSNESS

IT IS VERY difficult to sustain hope in devastating circumstances, especially during long-term care that may span years or even decades. Almost everyone in such situations experiences periods when despair takes over. You may feel overwhelmed and inadequate. When feelings of helplessness linger, depression is likely to develop. You may find yourself crying at odd times or sitting inert, unable to move.

For most people, having seven out of ten good days is considered "normal." But if you find yourself living under a constant dark cloud, your situation may have worn you down and you may be what is known as "situationally depressed." This kind of depression is not simply feeling sad. It is a sense of doom and gloom, and more night than light. It may be difficult to get out of bed, or once you are up and about, you may become unfocused and find it difficult to carry out everyday activities. You can even switch into what is known as "agitated depression," where you feel restless and filled with motor excitement, unable to stay still. Papers pile up, and perhaps tasks remain half finished. These feelings can be scary, and it's important to get help. If you feel yourself losing heart or becoming despondent, recognize these signs as a red flag. (See page 86 for further information on the symptoms of depression.)

Remember, you have a reason to feel blue. Events have sapped your energy, and it seems you are living your life in a fog. This is a time to reach out, get out of the house, or spend only limited time at the hospital or otherwise focused on your partner. Do something you love that is also good for you. Exercise and a heathy diet help. If you are too down to move, this is a perfect time to consider therapy and/or temporary medication. It's daunting to manage despair and hopelessness, but I've seen people do it and grow stronger.

GUILT

"WOULD THIS HAVE been avoided if I had taken him to the doctor on Monday instead of Wednesday?" a guilt-ridden wife asked when her husband was admitted to the hospital with internal bleeding. Wisely, the chief of the intensive care unit warned her, "Let's not go that route."

I call this the would have, could have, should have scenario. It beckons all who think there's something else they might have done to save their partner from harm. It is a version of magical thinking, where you view yourself as so powerful that you could have prevented this medical crisis. Guilt is also a reaction to experiencing helplessness. But bad things sometimes *do* happen to good people.

One woman can't forget how she snapped at her husband when she thought he was exaggerating his pain and "just looking for attention." In fact, he was terribly sick. "How could I have done that? He was ill."

Rachel can't forgive herself for a different reason. Her home-bound husband called her several times a day at work. She resented the interruptions and finally asked testily, "Why do you need to talk to me so much?" He proceeded to explain, "Don't you know it makes me feel closer to you? It comforts me to hear your voice."

"Why wasn't I more understanding?" she constantly asks herself. The answer is, she didn't know his real motivation. We all have moments we regret. But it does help to realize that when you're regularly annoyed at your mate, you probably need a break or at least some help. If you take care of yourself, you're far more likely to be patient with him.

Of course, there are also other manifestations of guilt. If he's in the hospital (or a nursing home) and your children take you out to a lovely restaurant for Mother's Day, you may feel pangs of guilt for having this special time for yourself. If your son is getting married and your mate can't attend the event, it can be difficult to allow yourself the fun of shopping for a dress. However, this is one of those times when you can't live your partner's pain. It doesn't help him if your day is spoiled.

Many people feel guilty and conflicted about putting their spouse in a nursing home. This is understandable. Sometimes as much as you love him, the burden of being a caregiver is just too much. You can't do it any longer. As hard as it may be to see him go to a nursing home, it may be better for both of you.

SEVEN WAYS TO HANDLE YOUR EMOTIONS

IT'S NORMAL TO experience a variety of negative emotions when your mate is seriously ill. The challenge is not to become mired in feelings that demoralize you. Here's how to cope.

1. Move past anxieties and fears.

Once you voice what you dread, you can look at the reality of the situation. After you say out loud, "I'm afraid he'll die," you can move on to, "How likely is it he will really die of this?" For example, the majority of men with prostate cancer will die of something else before this cancer kills them. Talk to the doctor and educate yourself about the facts, especially if you're someone who tends to panic and rush to the bottom line. Today many people live for decades with serious conditions that are managed.

If you say the words, "I'm afraid of being left alone," you can then look at how alone you really will be. You can ask, "Who are the people I can count on?" and even make a list of them. If there are few, this can be a wake-up call to start expanding your social circle and preparing for the future. What steps can you take to be less alone?

Just expressing the thought, "I'm afraid this will never end," can lighten your burden. Then you can examine the truth. Are you overreacting to a long stretch with no improvement—or do you indeed face years of caregiving ahead?

Jacqueline felt as if it was the end of the world when her husband became a total invalid for six weeks. "I was so discouraged. I thought he would never get better," she recalls. In fact, little by little he improved and finally did get out of bed.

On the other hand, if it is likely that he won't improve (or will worsen), it's time to plan. Someone with Alzheimer's may live anywhere from two to twenty years. That may affect a lot of decisions you make about hiring help—or joining a support group sooner rather than later.

2. Live in the moment.

The advice to "Take one day at a time" and "Live in the moment" has value. To live in the moment means to be fully present now, instead of worrying and wondering what will happen tomorrow, or next week, or next year. Maybe your partner will have a cancer recurrence in the future, but if you spend all of your time obsessing about it, you miss the pleasure of today.

"I used to sit at the hospital consumed by anxiety, wondering how I'd get through next week or next month," says one wife. "I was like a horse wearing blinders, shutting out anything that interfered with my worry. At some point, I finally gained the confidence to take one day (and sometimes one hour or one minute) at a time. That does get you through."

3. Try other anxiety-control strategies.

In my experience, anxiety is the most common feeling that spouse caregivers struggle with. Sometimes it is possible to reduce anxiety yourself. One of my clients found that when she woke up in the morning with a familiar tightening in her stomach, it helped to get up and have a cup of tea or coffee. "Just getting out of bed and walking to the kitchen helps a lot. That and setting up the coffee pot gets me involved. By the time I sit down at the table to drink a cup, the anxiety has usually faded or gone," she says.

Being vertical rather than horizontal seems to help most people. Staying prone in bed can leave you feeling powerless. Getting up and standing helps you feel more in control.

I also recommend to my clients these anxiety distracters—activities that absorb your attention and, in some cases, focus you: watching TV or videos; reading books or magazines; or listening to music. Also helpful are quiet or seemingly mindless activities that give a sense of satisfaction, such as peeling potatoes, ironing, rearranging drawers or closets, painting the bathroom, baking a cake, or weeding the garden. More proactive activities work well, too, such as visiting friends; taking care of children, grandchildren, or pets; exercising; volunteering to help others; becoming more involved in your place of worship; or becoming an activist for his disease or another cause you feel passionate about. Perhaps some of these ideas can work well for you.

4. Express anger appropriately.

Give yourself permission to have feelings of anger and even rage, which arise in many caregiving situations. Then you are less likely to explode. The goal is to find a way to express your feelings that won't hurt you or your mate while he's down.

Discuss your anger with a trusted friend or family member, a therapist, or in a support group where you can safely voice frustrations and shameful feelings toward your mate. It helps to know that other women have lost their temper with their mates, too. More than one person has wished the ordeal would end.

After Rachel returned from her first support group meeting, her husband was so thrilled with the change in her that he urged her to attend anytime. Rachel said of her experience: "In the group I was able to get out all my anger at his neediness. By the time I got home, I felt filled with love for him. I kept hugging and kissing him." Expressing her negative feelings freed her to feel all the deep, loving ones. And he basked in the burst of attention.

5. Beware of stoicism.

Stoicism is the appearance of being unaffected by what you are feeling. You seem impassive and unmoved by joy or grief. Too often I see clients who try to be stoic during a mate's illness. Almost without exception, they pay a heavy price for suppressing their emotions. Their feelings leak out in the form of physical symptoms or illnesses.

I once treated a captain in the U.S. Navy whose husband of fifteen years lay in a coma. She used denial and stoicism as a defense against the reality of the situation—and said she came to me only because the navy insisted she get help, not because she needed it.

She kept repeating, "I'm fine," in an almost robotic way. Yet she had developed colitis, and a rash that appeared all over her body at different times of the day and night. As we talked, this stoic woman soon began to sob. Words tumbled out along with her tears, and together we watched an amazing reaction. Her rash started to fade.

This seemingly magical cure may be hard to believe at first. It is easier to understand when you realize how closely the mind, body, and spirit interconnect. I believe the rash represented feelings she had never expressed, which were trapped beneath her skin. It makes sense that the strong emotions you keep inside may emerge in annoying ways. For the captain, it was the rash. Metaphorically, she had something under her skin. For others, it's headaches, stomachaches, or serious illness. We know that shingles can be related to stress and can appear at difficult times.

People often function well during the day and then wake up in the middle of the night with palpitations and panic attacks. Or they blow up at someone who doesn't deserve it, or kick the dog. If you're one of these people, there's a better way. Getting feelings out of your system appropriately is a little like emptying a clogged kitchen drain. It clears the blockage and allows you to function again.

It breaks your heart to see the person you love so sick. You're allowed to cry if you feel sad, as Yi Ping does. "I go downstairs, sit on the sofa, and let the tears roll out for a while. Then I pick myself up and go back up. I feel better," she says.

A good cry together with your mate—and yes, some men do cry—can help you share your pain as a couple. It is a reminder that you are a team. Just be careful that shedding tears together doesn't become a "bond of the blues" where you both descend into a downward spiral.

6. **Acknowledge the upside: positive emotions.**

I believe most people have a remarkable amount of resilience. You not only can grow through desperate times, but you also can transform and transcend. In the process, you have the opportunity to experience pride in what you accomplish, in mastery of tasks you never thought you could do, in overcoming fear of failure, and you may possibly achieve transformational love. Allow yourself to acknowledge these positive emotions. They balance the difficult challenges you face and become a steadying force. Congratulate yourself on the new skills you've learned.

On the other hand, others' expectations that they *should* feel positive can drive some women nuts. They find no personal fulfillment in caregiving. If you fall into this category, be true to yourself. No one can be up all the time.

7. Write a letter.

I often ask clients to write a letter to their mate that is never mailed instead of obsessing about an upset. It's a way to find out what you really feel and often satisfies your need to express yourself without risking unnecessary confrontation. A typical letter to your partner might read something like, "Dear Jack, I love you beyond belief, but I want you to know that sometimes you make me angry." Writing has an advantage over speaking to him, because although your unconscious anger may leak through, an unmailed letter is safe. You can say, "I couldn't stand you today" on paper, and nobody gets hurt.

NAVIGATING
EMOTIONAL SHOALS

PEOPLE OFTEN KEEP their most private pain to themselves. But if you talk (or write) about feelings that are the most troubling to you, you can cut them down to size and decide whether you need help and what kind.

I know that acknowledging your feelings is easier said than done, especially when you're feeling lost and alone. Try to be kind to yourself as you move through this necessary process. I often tell my clients, "More curiosity, less judgment." By this I mean, try to wonder what is happening and why. When assaulted by difficult issues, rushing to the bottom line hurts both of you.

Reflections

- *No matter how inadequate you may feel, you are your partner's most important support.*

- *Almost everyone in your situation feels the way you do at one time or another. You are not alone.*

- *Instead of burying your feelings, express them—but do it appropriately.*

- *Don't judge yourself harshly. It doesn't help you or your partner. Have more curiosity and less judgment.*

- *Live in the present; you can't change the past. Forgive yourself.*

14

Making Your Needs
a Priority

Research shows a strong relationship between taking
care of an ill or disabled family member and a decline in the caregiver's health. The link is particularly strong if the patient is your
mate. Caregivers can also be prone to accidents. If you're overwhelmed, anxious, or depressed, you aren't focused. One woman
scalded her arm with steaming coffee. Another got caught in elevator doors. Some trip in the street because they aren't paying
attention.

It's hard to notice the crack in the sidewalk if you're wondering why his medication won't work, how you'll manage after he's
home from the hospital, or whether the aide will show up today.
When most of your attention centers on his needs, your own
well-being ranks way down on the list of priorities.

You can't afford *not* to take care of yourself—for his sake as
much as your own. If you catch the flu, break an ankle, or sink
into depression, who will be there for him? In order to protect
your health, you have the right to say yes to your own priorities.

HOW ARE *YOU*?

AS YOU TAKE care of your partner during his illness, are you also taking your own health needs seriously? To gauge how well (or how poorly) you take care of yourself during this stressful time, check True or False for the statements below.

1. I feel exhausted much of the time.

   _____ True   _____ False

2. It's hard for me to concentrate.

   _____ True   _____ False

3. At times I feel as if I'm drowning.

   _____ True   _____ False

4. I don't have enough support from others.

   _____ True   _____ False

5. I often have trouble sleeping.

   _____ True   _____ False

6. Lately I get sick easily.

   _____ True   _____ False

7. I feel blue and have no appetite (or overeat).

   _____ True   _____ False

8. I have a short fuse and flare up easily.

   _____ True   _____ False

9. I seem to have more than my share of accidents.

_____ True   _____ False

10. I haven't had fun in a very long time.

_____ True   _____ False

11. I haven't seen a doctor for myself in over a year.

_____ True   _____ False

12. I have a serious medical condition.

_____ True   _____ False

13. I do not attend a support group, see a therapist, or talk to a friend or relative about my troubles.

_____ True   _____ False

14. I have no time for my own needs.

_____ True   _____ False

15. I rarely ask for help or use community resources.

_____ True   _____ False

If you checked True for five or more of these statements, you are not making your health and well-being a priority and are putting yourself at risk.

PAY ATTENTION TO YOUR HEALTH ISSUES

"HOW CAN I go to the doctor about a mole that's probably nothing when he's so ill?" This kind of thinking is a common excuse for putting your own health last. You may even believe that your partner is the only legitimate recipient of care—that you don't count. The question is, How can you not see the dermatologist when your man is depending on you? Your own doctor visits are just as important as his. Resist the temptation to postpone or break them—for his sake, as well as your own.

Serious Risks

Are you overweight or inactive? Do you have high blood pressure or high cholesterol? If any of these are true for you, pay attention. These are risk factors for health problems. Diabetes, heart disease, and arthritis may become issues as you get older, and your medications may need monitoring. Also, once you pass fifty, you're more likely to be diagnosed with breast cancer. After fifty-five, risk of stroke doubles every decade.

One wife with a strong family history of heart disease and diabetes realized that she was so engrossed in her husband's health problems that she hadn't had a physical in four years. "I used to depend on my gynecologist to check everything, but he changed his office practice and stopped doing that. I realized that I had to take charge and make an appointment with an internist. The wake-up call was my friend's sudden heart attack. She's six years younger than I am."

Sleep Deprivation

Another health risk that is linked to the role of taking care of a sick partner is lack of sleep. A good night's rest is your body's way of refueling, but when your mate is ill, sleep can be elusive for a number of reasons. The dark hours of night are prime time for worry and obsessing. You may toss and turn while ruminating about his condition. Or he may wake you up at three a.m. to help him go to the bathroom. Or perhaps a part of you always remains on high alert listening to see if he is still breathing. "I was anxious all the time because I didn't know what was coming. For a year and a half I was so tuned in to him I was up all night. It wasn't until we got the defibrillator that I slept through," says Hannah, whose husband has a heart condition.

Whatever the cause, there's no question that loss of sleep leaves you fatigued and exhausted. It interferes with clear thinking, judgment, and your ability to absorb information. Lack of sleep may slow your reaction time, increase anxiety, and make you more irritable.

Imagine sleepless nights going on for four years, as they did for Marjorie, whose husband suffered from dementia. He would get up at midnight, decide it was daytime, and dress up in a suit and tie, insisting he had to go to a meeting. "It took me awhile to figure out how to deal with it. I would tell him, 'The meeting is tomorrow. You're a day early.' Then I'd get him undressed and back into bed. One night he got dressed again an hour later. It was so exhausting," recalls Marjorie, who paid a heavy toll in weight loss and other physical symptoms. Eventually, she had to hire help.

On the other hand, if worry becomes insomnia, this may be a time for medication. It's best to talk with your doctor about a prescription for a sleep medication that doesn't have next-day side effects. Some over-the-counter sleep aids may help as well, but many can leave you groggy the next morning. Check with a medical professional before you self-medicate. People often feel embarrassed to discuss sleep problems with a physician, but such issues are too important to ignore.

THE SHADOW OF DEPRESSION

IN THE GENERAL population, twice as many women as men suffer from depression. It makes sense that you're even more susceptible to depression when your husband is sick, especially if the illness is chronic.

Beware, however, of a common message in our society that depression is your fault. Some people believe that if you simply think positive thoughts, all will be well. That is not necessarily true. In dealing with a mate's illness, depression can be a realistic reaction to overwhelming stress. Don't suffer in silence. Get help.

It takes effort to try to be serene and compassionate all of the time—effort you can't afford on top of daily tasks and responsibilities. A client of mine put it this way: "I get really depressed when people say I should think positively about my husband's condition. I feel like telling the person, 'Of course I try to think positively, but day to day my feelings are all over the place. Sometimes I'm so angry I have to walk out of the room because I want to smack him when his demands get too much for me. I love him dearly, but I'm human, too. There's only so much I can do."

This woman echoes a statement I often hear from caregivers. They are frayed at the edges and scared. Few of us can control our emotions at all times or be perfect healers, nor should we try to be. For further information on depression, see pages 85–87, 96–97 and 223–224.

THE ROLE OF THERAPY

THE ORIGINAL MEANING of psychotherapy comes from the Greek word "psyche," or soul, and therapists were considered healers. They can be healers today, too. There are times when professional help is necessary to deal with issues such as your sense of loss, unresolved anger, or depression. Sometimes medication is part of the equation to allow you to function and help you get through the most difficult days. A combination of therapy and prescribed medication helped Marjorie, the woman whose husband got dressed at midnight. She also attended a support group.

Another woman, deeply religious, whose husband has suffered from multiple sclerosis for years, observes, "I've needed therapy and medication to take care of my primary organ, the brain, and I feel our creator would be in favor of that. It made all the difference in my ability to cope. Some people think therapy means they're weak and don't have strength. It takes great courage to ask for help."

Florence believes she couldn't have survived her husband's bouts of illness without therapy. "I'm not entirely sure why it works, but it does for me. I walk in trembling with anxiety and feeling trapped, and I pour out my worst nightmares. A day or two later, things start to look different. I see options that seemed impossible before," she says.

Not just any therapist will do, of course. Therapy is divided into multiple schools of thought. Be aware that different therapists have different orientations. Some will help you specifically with your immediate problems. Some will offer only medication or techniques such as behavior modification. Others take a broader view and will help you look at yourself, your relationships, and your view of life. If you have an unsatisfactory experience in therapy—and if after discussing what bothers you with the therapist you don't get an acceptable response—remember, you are the boss and can walk out. Don't let one negative incident stop you from looking elsewhere. There are many methods and many kinds of practitioners. When choosing one, make sure you connect with the person and feel understood. You're going to talk about intimate issues, such as emotional pain and sorrow, and you have to feel comfortable. Even in a low-cost clinic or a facility attached to a training institute or university or hospital, some professionals are better for you than others. Without a good therapeutic relationship and a sense of trust, it's hard for a person to change.

Look for someone who is empathetic and who knows the complexities of your situation. Ask around. A good place to start is the organization relevant to your partner's disease, which is likely to maintain a list of experienced professionals who are known to be effective.

THE ROLE OF SPIRITUALITY

Spirituality or faith is a powerful resource that you carry within you. In the 1950s, Helen Keller said in Edward R. Murrow's series *This I Believe,* "By faith I mean a vision of good one cherishes and enthusiasm that pushes one to seek its fulfillment regardless of obstacles. . . . Faith invigorates the will, enriches the affections, and awakens a sense of creativeness." Faith puts you in touch with your soul and helps you focus on healing, comfort, renewal, and self-acceptance. Many people find that a deep faith helps them cope with the stress of taking care of a sick mate, as well as any illness of their own.

Although spirituality or faith often takes the form of rituals and religious belief, it can also refer to enhancing the human spirit through other practices. One path is to connect with nature. Mountain and sky, water or woods, the sway of a tulip—all of these link us with something larger than ourselves. Research suggests that contact with the great outdoors can nurture the soul and improve your health and well-being. Fortunately, you don't necessarily have to go far. You can find nature by strolling in a local park. You need the exercise, which also increases your endorphins and makes you feel better. Nature lives, too, in a backyard garden or even a window box. If nature is not for you, other spiritual experiences include quiet reflection while walking city streets, or enjoying the beauty of art in a museum.

The Power of Belief

Many studies also show that religious affiliation and prayer, which is only one expression of spirituality, are associated with better health and longer life and seem to have a positive effect on cardiovascular and immune function. For those who believe "God doesn't give me more than I can handle," religious benefits can include stress relief. Hannah explains, "People often ask, 'How can you take care of him when he's so sick?' I say, 'God keeps me going.'" Others find comfort in believing "There's a reason things happen. Bad times make us stronger."

Another woman attends seven a.m. Mass every morning while her husband is still sleeping. "I do a lot of praying and say, 'Dear God, here it is. You've got to help me through this day.'" The act of centering herself and putting herself in the hands of a higher power helps sustain her.

SPIRITUALITY AND COMPLEMENTARY OR ALTERNATIVE MEDICINE

MANY PEOPLE FIND complementary or alternative medicine (CAM) useful. Some practices have a spiritual component. Sixty-two percent of adults use CAM approaches, including prayer, and the National Center for Complementary and Alternative Medicine (NCCAM) is now a part of the National Institutes of Health.

CAM is an increasingly popular resource for those with chronic conditions. For example, a doctor may recommend massage therapy or acupuncture to reduce the inflammation and pain of arthritis. Yoga can help reduce stiffness, fatigue, anxiety, and depression.

In diabetics, yoga improves immune function and can help control blood sugar. It also lowers blood pressure and has many other therapeutic effects.

Meditation can reduce anxiety, pain, blood pressure, and depression. Guided imagery, a technique of focused relaxation, brings serenity and helps you feel grounded . An example is to envision a calm image, such as a beautiful, peaceful pond, and find tranquility. We all can recall scenes that aid us in reconnecting with our core. Biofeedback, hypnosis, reflexology, and chiropractic are among other options.

Sometimes homeopathic treatments seem to help when conventional medications do not. However, be sure to check out herbal medications, vitamins, and minerals with your doctor before trying them (and inform him or her of any you already take). These can have dangerous interactions with prescribed drugs, such as some heart medications.

Strong beliefs and the structure of ritual pulled Lea through her husband's multiple health crises. When anxiety threatened to overwhelm her, she called on her faith to calm her down. "I was very nervous when he needed several prostate and back surgeries. I prayed and meditated during each operation. I also have a strong church family right by my side. There was only one point when I went to pieces, and the preacher visited the day I fell apart. Without him, I don't know what I would have done. Just having him there was a help in case something happened," she recalls.

However, some people react differently. They rage at God for abandoning them and allowing catastrophe to strike. This kind of response can be emotionally useful, allowing them to rant, rave, and feel more powerful. It may even strengthen their negotiating skills. Some people turn to God; some turn away; others vacillate along their journey. There is no right path.

Of course you want to do your best for your partner, but that's usually not possible unless you refresh your spirit with or without religious faith. It may not be easy to get in touch with your spiritual self if it has never been important in your life. Yet it is possible to explore that part of you now and find solace.

SEVEN WAYS TO MAKE SURE YOUR HEALTH MATTERS, TOO

WE KNOW THAT your mate's health problems make a significant impact on your own mental and physical well-being. Under stress, your immune system is compromised. Here are some suggestions for staying as strong as possible:

1. Pace yourself to conserve energy.

When a client of mine was on a respirator and sedated in the intensive care unit for two weeks, the doctor told his wife, "Don't hang around here. Save your energy and rest. Later, he'll want you present all the time." He gave her permission to take care of herself, and she did. Monique visited her husband every day at the hospital but didn't stay long.

"I'd talk to him for a while, but there was no response, of course, and I couldn't keep it up. It dragged me down to spend too much time there. The doctor was right. After my husband was moved to a regular room, he wanted me there constantly. I was ready," says Monique.

There may also be physical tasks at home that wear you out. Your back is probably going to suffer if your mate must be lifted in and out of a bed or wheelchair. If you can't afford help, perhaps a willing neighbor might assist. A caregiver class may be useful, too. (See page 35.)

The stress of caregiving can overwhelm you in diagnoses such as stroke, hip fracture, congestive heart failure, and dementia. Such dramatic impairment places a tremendous burden on you. Don't let it make you sick or lead you to take out your feelings on your mate.

2. **Recognize resistance to help.**

Some people have sufficient help when caring for an ill mate, but many others don't. According to Rev. Elizabeth Eisen:

Often people who say they're "just fine" live in a bubble of self-sufficiency and believe needing help is a sign of weakness. They try to trudge on alone. Others are convinced they are the only ones who can take proper care of him and won't allow themselves even an hour or two away. Understand how important it is to take care of yourself and have your own life. You have that right. If you're just plain too tired to get yourself out the door to go someplace else for a meeting, rest a little at home, then call someone. "I almost didn't come tonight" is often heard at support group meetings. Getting to the meeting does take extra effort, but once there, participants realize that connecting with others energizes rather than depletes them.

At first, Monique refused to get extra help when her husband came home from the hospital with multiple health issues, even though they could afford assistance. Soon she reversed her thinking. "I felt trapped and exhausted, and my husband and I were so scared, we were at each other's throats. I balked at the intrusion of having a private aide in our apartment, but at the urging of my children, I finally gave in and hired one. It freed me to go out whenever I wanted, and even to go away once overnight," she recalls.

3. Get enough sleep.

Inez had a tough year when complications of diabetes kept sending her physicist husband to the hospital: "I realized that when I went to bed every night, I felt such stress that my body barely lay on top of the mattress in anticipation of jumping up at the slightest sound or movement that didn't seem normal. Instead of sinking into the pillow top, I felt like an ironing board on the bed. Two things finally helped me get to sleep: (1) Inhaling very slowly to a count of ten or twelve and exhaling to that same count. The counting itself is relaxing; and (2) Reciting the Lord's Prayer over and over again like a mantra." Relaxation techniques can help you, too.

If your mate has dementia or Alzheimer's disease, do what new parents and many caregivers do: when he takes a nap, you take a nap. According to the National Institutes of Health, a short nap of up to an hour can help compensate for lost sleep the night before. No naps after three p.m., however, or they may interfere with nighttime sleep. I have recommended that clients ask (or hire) someone to sleep over at times if that is the only way they can get a night's rest.

If it's worry that robs you of sleep, here are some things you can do:

- Avoid lying awake in bed for an extended period of time. Get up and read a book until you feel drowsy.
- Go to sleep at the same time every night.
- Get out in sunlight for at least thirty minutes a day.
- Avoid caffeine, alcohol, and big meals before bed.
- Be aware that certain medications may affect sleep, such as some drugs for high blood pressure, heart disease, and asthma.

If you continue to have a problem, talk with your doctor. Remember, chronic sleep deprivation increases your risk of depression.

4. Beware of other signs of stress and burnout.

One wife knew she'd reached the brink of burnout when she forgot her handbag in a restaurant, then left it on a store counter and again in a taxi in the space of two weeks. Car accidents and falls are also common when you're distracted. If strange things are happening to you, you're sending yourself a message to take heed of your own needs—or else.

Know your body. For example, heart palpitations can be a sign of overwhelming stress. Overeating and not eating are both signals, too. You may have lost your appetite (or even feel nauseous much of the time) in response to stress or because you're depressed. Realize that food is fuel. Make sure you don't miss meals.

On the other hand, you don't want to turn to the refrigerator and grab everything in sight. Hannah, who is at risk for stroke herself, wound up eating healthier as a result of her husband's diet regimen. "I had to learn a new way to cook and eat, because he couldn't have salt or too much fat. When he came home from the hospital, the dietician gave him a 'budget' of how much he could have. He made a chart and recorded what he ate for three months. It helped both of us. I ate what he ate, because it was healthy and I had to be healthy, too."

Ironically, your partner may be in better shape than you are. He sees physicians all the time. You're the one who cancels doctor's appointments again and again.

5. Schedule in physical activity.

Not all personality types do best with conventional relaxation techniques to cope with stress. If you're someone whose energy seems to need physical outlets, try exercise. Florence hopped on the treadmill or worked out with weights and did abdominal exercises to take her mind off her husband's condition. Even at the worst times, she always felt stronger and more centered afterward. It is well known that exercise effectively fights depression.

Yoga in various forms has become the single most popular stress-relieving activity in this country, and it increases energy, too. And don't forget other possibilities, such as running or fast walking, Pilates, and martial arts, such as tai chi, which improves balance, increases strength, and can significantly reduce the risk of falls. Learn what your body responds to and do what helps.

6. **Try expressive writing.**

Keep a journal and write regularly about your thoughts and feelings regarding your mate's illness and how it has affected your life. Write in a free-flowing, stream of consciousness fashion, without judgment and censorship, and get it all out—the good, the bad, and the ugly. Writing about disturbing events gets your thoughts and feelings out of your system and has significant health benefits. It can boost your immune system, reduce asthma and arthritis symptoms, lower blood pressure, and even reduce visits to the doctor. The therapeutic benefit may have to do with gaining insight, changing the way you look at what has happened, and increasing self-esteem.

Writing in your journal can be especially helpful when you have ambivalent feelings, such as love and resentment, that can coexist when you fear your mate will never be the same. It can clear the path to figure out what to do and how to do it. If you write down, "I don't *want* to go to the hospital today. I can't stand it," you might then think about calling your sister-in-law and asking her to stand in for you.

7. Give yourself a break.

One wife who spends twenty-four hours a day with her husband told me, "It's such a bother to put him in day care or ask someone to stay with him while I get away. It's easier just to stay home." That's often a handy but bogus excuse (and can be a sign of depression).

Everyone needs time off to refuel, to catch up on sleep and everything else. If a friend invites you out for lunch or dinner or away for the weekend, go, even though you may feel anxious while you're away. If your partner protests the idea of your spending time away from him, don't let it stop you. Time off is actually a relationship saver. You return refreshed and more alive (not to mention more patient), and bring back experiences to share that energize your marriage.

Perhaps there are times when you experience feelings of desperation. You've had enough and must get away for more than a few hours. If you can afford it, get someone to cover for you and go to a hotel for a night—or take your friend up on her offer of the extra bedroom. You're not a deserter, just a very tired woman in great need.

Take advantage of community programs that give you a break. For example, respite care offers temporary substitute care for your mate (at home or in another location), which allows you to take a day, weekend, or longer period off for vacation. If your partner is sixty or over, an adult day care center provides social, recreational, and health-related services. Eldercare Locator, a national directory of community services, can help you find local programs online at www.eldercare.gov, or call 800-677-1116.

THE ART OF SELF-PRESERVATION

THERE IS ALWAYS a pull between your needs and his. You may well ask, "How can I take time to put on my sneakers and fast-walk for forty minutes or make an appointment with the eye doctor? How can I go away for the weekend?" But there's a difference between healthy self-care and selfishness, although people often confuse the two.

Constantly putting yourself last not only hurts you, it can increase the likelihood you'll behave negatively toward your mate. To help keep your own well-being on your radar screen, you might want to try a system of rewards, an idea one of my clients used successfully. She gave herself a fifteen-minute reward to relax and stretch out, eat, and otherwise tend to her own needs for every hour she engaged in tasks for her husband. This was her way to continue to be a good caregiver and also take care of herself.

Reflections

- Get enough rest. You can't run on empty.

- Beware of your own protests that you're fine.

- If you're spiritual, take comfort in your faith, prayer, or nature, whatever speaks to your soul.

- Eat healthily, schedule physical activity, or find other ways to improve your well-being.

- Remember, taking good care of yourself is smart, not selfish.

15

When Doing Your Best
Is Not Enough

"Grief is the price we pay for love," said Queen Elizabeth II. Sometimes, no matter what you do, no matter how effective you are, no matter how much you love him, your efforts are simply not enough. Your worst nightmare comes true. Your mate suddenly collapses on the golf course, or his death becomes inevitable after a fatal diagnosis or a long illness. He is going to die in weeks or months, not years, and the reality staggers both your heart and mind. As you begin a journey of anguish and enormous change, you may feel certain that you'll never recover. Yet there are ways to find meaning in what lies ahead.

Over the years, I've helped clients negotiate this most devastating life transition. With emotional, spiritual, and practical assistance (and not without great difficulty), many have grown in ways they never anticipated. They've found a measure of peace and the courage to move on. That is my wish for you.

THE GIFT OF TIME

A DEATH THAT comes suddenly is one of the most difficult to process. The shock is so great. There is no chance to absorb what has happened, to adjust, or say good-bye. But if you and your partner have the gift of time, you have an opportunity to help him prepare for his death—and learn to let go yourself. It's a painful process to accept what must be, even when you know nothing else can be done. This is true even when you believe in an afterlife and that he is going to a better place. I hope to make this transition a more meaningful, enriching experience for both of you.

The term "dying well" is a relatively recent concept in our society, although the idea has always been part of Native American and certain other cultures. When I refer to dying well, I mean helping your mate live through this period as comfortably as possible—physically, emotionally, and spiritually. Now is the time to try to maximize his quality of life in every way. Although a complete cure is no longer on the table, relief of pain and symptoms (palliative care) usually is. In today's world, dying does not have to mean terrible suffering.

At the same time, dying is more than a collection of symptoms. Although usually surrounded by grief and sorrow, it is also a continuation of the life cycle. Substantial growth can occur, because dying well embraces the whole range of human experience, including dealing with the greatest fear most of us have—fear of death. Many couples I've worked with have been able to deepen their relationship during this time.

RESPECTING YOUR PARTNER'S WISHES

"I WANTED TO be with him every minute of this precious time. I loved him more each day," says Norah. This last period brought her and her husband, Patrick, an architect in his fifties, closer together. Patrick suddenly received a diagnosis of advanced melanoma after what was supposed to be a routine test. They were told he had six months to live. Norah made the decision to leave her job to devote herself to him for the time they had left. Her dedication enabled Patrick, a strong, silent type who was distant to many people, to become more expressive. He was able to find the words to tell Norah how deeply he loved her.

As they faced his death, they cried together. They talked about the children, their home, their travels, and all the memories that had brought them joy. They also used the time they had left to plan realistically for the future. Patrick had a large life insurance policy, and they decided that Norah would spend part of the proceeds to pay off their mortgage. This would allow Norah and the children to remain in their home. Patrick told her he wanted her to be happy and hoped she'd remarry. In turn, she talked about how much she would miss him and how he would always remain in her heart.

Not every couple negotiates this ultimate transition so smoothly. For an Omaha couple, Toni and Gil, it became a rocky time. Their marriage began to deteriorate after Gil, a bank executive, was diagnosed with kidney cancer and given less than a year to live. He reacted by changing significantly in ways that made life difficult for Toni and their two young children. Gil made a bargain with God, promising he would become more devout if God would save him. He became obsessed with finding a cure, trying all kinds of diets and traveling to clinics abroad.

Some people don't accept that death is inevitable, and this is not necessarily a bad thing. However, Gil's desperation and self-centeredness led Toni to feel resentful. He constantly yelled at the children and insisted Toni leave a part-time accounting job she loved. "I needed to get out of the house. My office was five minutes from home. But I couldn't say no to him, because he was dying." Although the couple attended counseling together, they couldn't connect except for times when Gil would periodically break down and apologize. Then they would hug and cry.

It is ultimately healing to feel the sadness, sorrow, and pain of impending death. Hopefully, you can reach acceptance and peace together. This kind of coping is very hard to do, because your partner is scared and angry that he is dying, and you are scared and angry that he is leaving.

Marriages have different strengths and weaknesses, as we all do. The couple Toni and Gil were a mixed bag. They loved each other and were very functional and task oriented, but they needed more help with processing their feelings. Yet they did leave a legacy of their life together. They had made plans to renovate their house before Gil's diagnosis.

"It sounds nutty, but we went ahead with it," Toni recalls. "We added a whole new wing. It was like therapy to pick out furniture and tile, and we actually finished it before he died. Working together on the project helped us bear the stress, and it got me out." In a way, the renovation was Gil's last gift to Toni, a gift that speaks to the future.

Toni did the best she could to deal with a very difficult husband in trying circumstances. She continued therapy on her own to help her make peace with all that happened.

THE FIVE STAGES OF GRIEF

IN HER BOOK *On Death and Dying,* the late psychiatrist Elisabeth Kübler-Ross identified five stages through which the dying come to terms with death:

1. Denial: He says, "This isn't happening to me," and acts as if his life will go on forever.

2. Anger: He asks, "Why is this happening to me?" Sometimes he rails against everyone, including God.

3. Bargaining: He promises he'll do anything if he doesn't have to die—be a better husband, father, or friend.

4. Depression: He reluctantly begins to give in to the inevitable. He thinks or says, "I don't care anymore" (often accompanied by a sense of helplessness and hopelessness).

5. Acceptance: He feels relaxed, ready to let go, and at peace with whatever comes.

Kübler-Ross identified the five stages in a particular order, but mental health professionals now believe there is no exact script and that people experience these stages in a zigzag fashion. They can bounce from one stage to another in their own individual way, or even skip a stage, like Gil, who never got to acceptance.

PLANNING TOGETHER, IF POSSIBLE

THE TRANSITION FROM life to death can feel like a time of ultimate helplessness. All roads have been closed; there is no escape. However, there may be a surprising number of choices available throughout the process, unless his condition makes it impossible for him to consider them. It is easier to cope and make essential decisions if you can talk together openly about these questions:

How does he feel about medical intervention?

Issues concerning medical intervention are difficult to think about and discuss, but what if his heart stops? What should you do? It's best not to assume what he wants, because you may be wrong. Does he want to be resuscitated? One man did, although hospital personnel tried to persuade him to change his mind. His sentiment was, "You do the best you can." Others feel differently. How about a ventilator? Does he want a feeding tube? One man was too frightened to make these decisions.

The best thing to do is something many people shy away from—have advance directives ready which say, "This is how I want to die." Advance directives are legal documents that provide instructions about an individual's future medical care if the person cannot speak for himself or herself. It is important that your mate create these documents, because they allow you to act as he would want and make stressful decisions about his health care so much easier. They include:

- **Health Care Proxy (or Durable Power of Attorney for Health Care)**—This names someone (probably you) to make health care decisions in accordance with his wishes and to interpret his wishes. The proxy can be used whether or not he is terminally ill.

- **Living Will**—When he can no longer express what he wants, this details his wishes regarding his care and treatment. It is used only if he is terminal and has less than six months to live, is permanently unconscious, or is otherwise unable to make his own medical decisions.

  Both the health care proxy and living will vary from state to state. You can download free forms for your state at the National Hospice and Palliative Care Web site, www.caringinfo.org, or call 800-658-8898.

- **Do Not Resuscitate Order (DNR)**—A doctor must write this order as part of your advance directive. This is something you can plan ahead for.

Advance directives can be a difficult subject to broach, but you can take a deep breath and try. You can say, "Honey, can we fill out this form together?" Be prepared that he may reply, "Just do it."

What if you disagree with him? Supposedly the final say is his, but families don't always listen. One high-level executive couldn't let her husband go even though he gave instructions to do so. Sometimes there are conflicting wishes, but I believe his desires should prevail.

Where does he want to die?

Most people want to die in their own home. If that's possible, hospice care can be a tremendous help. *Hospice* is an umbrella term for programs that help the terminally ill prepare for death with dignity. These programs, which accept people who are expected to die within six months, are designed to enhance the person's quality of life and to ease his or her mental and physical suffering. Care includes pain control, symptom management, and psychological counseling, and in most cases takes place at home, although it can be at a hospice center. Medical personnel, home aides, social workers, and others work with the patient and family.

Hospice is covered by Medicare and by most private insurance. You can locate a program in your area along with other helpful information at the National Hospice and Palliative Care Organization Web site, www.caringinfo.org, or call 800-658-8898.

Would he like spiritual support?

Gil found solace by immersing himself in his religion. Even if your mate has not been religious before, he may feel differently now and may want to speak with a member of the clergy. Spiritual questions often arise when death is on the horizon. People wonder about going to heaven, an afterlife, even reincarnation. Past transgressions may weigh on their conscience.

One man, a Roman Catholic, always attended his wife's Protestant church. She wished a priest had come over when he was dying and had asked her husband if he wanted to take communion. She muses, "I think that would have been important to him. I bought a Bible and read psalms to him, and he liked that a lot, but because I'm not Catholic, I felt inadequate." In such situations, you can ask your mate directly whether he wants spiritual guidance or rituals. You can say, "Would you like to see a priest? Do you want last rites?" If he can't communicate, try to do what you think he wants.

Chaplains and other personnel are trained to offer both religious and spiritual help in hospitals and hospice. Many patients need this support. One hospital chaplain told me, "It doesn't matter what religion the patient is, because religion is about how you find your God—and this is about spirituality. I do stay aware and respectful of the person's faith, but we all share the same hopes and desires. We all can reflect and take steps toward hope and reconciliation. Many people of other religions say, 'Pray for me.'"

Does he want to see people?

Some people have been able to strengthen bonds with children, siblings, and others they love, and create moments of meaning as death approaches. They may even reconcile with people they've cut off. Others want privacy, not visitors. They don't want to be seen in decline.

For example, much of his community wanted to say good-bye to Patrick, the architect. He couldn't tolerate being seen in a compromised position and wanted to be remembered as the strong man he had been. He socialized with no one and bonded only with his wife, Norah, and his nurse. He stayed in the bedroom when people visited Norah, which was hard on her and everyone else who loved him.

Norah, on the other hand, who lost thirty pounds during this period, needed the love and support of others. She couldn't have helped Patrick without it. Friends brought food every day and assisted in other ways, allowing her to be with him continuously during those last weeks. Even though he denied the community, the community came to her.

What funeral and burial arrangements does he want?

After learning he had a few months to live, one man asked his wife to drive with him to look at cemetery plots. They found one in a pretty spot and decided he would be buried there. Someone else asked to be buried in New Mexico on a hill next to his parents and sister.

Does your mate want to be cremated? One man wanted his ashes shot into space. Others want them flung into a lake or the ocean.

Some people want to plan their funeral. Others don't *want* a funeral. They want a memorial service, a celebration, or a quiet gathering. There are so many possibilities.

WHEN YOUR PARTNER WON'T TALK

THE PRECEDING INSIGHTS become less useful when your mate is someone who refuses to talk about dying and its many details. Some people don't even want to know their prognosis. If this is the situation with your partner, you may feel torn about respecting his wishes.

Sarabeth faced this challenge when her husband, Larry, a construction foreman, became progressively weaker with an untreatable lung disease. He was told he had a year at most to live. Although both Larry and Sarabeth knew he was dying, he did not want to talk about it or even hear the word "death." He told his parents and siblings that nothing could be done, period.

Nevertheless, Sarabeth and their daughter felt that they should discuss his condition with him. They first checked with his doctor, who discouraged the idea. He told them, "If you talk to him about dying, he'll be dead in two weeks. He's a fighter and that's the way he wants it." Agreeing with this reasoning, Sarabeth dropped the idea.

Larry handled his illness the way he lived—by keeping an upbeat outlook and talking positively about the future. In such cases, this is not the time to try to alter his personality. You may help him, lead him, or show him, but don't try to push him. As in the story of Patrick, there are ways a man facing death may change. But it's unrealistic to expect a major shift in who he has always been.

Behaving Lovingly

If you know death is coming, you can deal with it in the most loving way possible whether or not he communicates openly. Both of you will gain. Try to take every opportunity to be intimate, respectful, and affectionate. Tell him every day that you love him. Bring him that unasked-for cup of water. Make his favorite food if he can eat, wear his favorite dress to give him pleasure, play his favorite music, touch him as you pass. There is little that substitutes for a caring caress.

When Patrick could no longer speak, Norah sat by his bedside stroking his hand. She talked with him about their life together. Norah understood that he was clinging to life for her. She gave him permission to go. "I'll be okay," she told him. Such kind, loving behavior doesn't mean you don't cry, but you can combine tears with reassurance that you will go on. Such reassurance can bring your partner solace, and you may benefit as well.

PREPARING CHILDREN FOR DAD'S DEATH

TONI AND GIL were able to talk openly about his cancer. "That was good for the kids. They knew what was going on and knew that some people died from this," says Toni.

Gil died at midnight on a Saturday night in the hospital, after Toni made a 911 call. His young sons slept through the arrival of the ambulance, and a friend stayed overnight with them. The next morning Toni told her oldest son, "Daddy got really sick last night and he died." She recalls, "He looked at me and said, 'Daddy is with the angels. He's not going to hurt anymore. If he gets a paper cut, it's not going to hurt. Can I watch TV?'"

This boy's quick shift from squarely facing his father's death to focusing on his favorite television program touches me. It's so typical of the way many children cope with the loss of a loved one. Young children live in the moment, and often their symptoms of grieving appear indirectly. They may seem fine at first and may not shed a tear. However, they may suddenly balk at going to school, eat more or less than usual, experience changes in sleep patterns, cling, or shut themselves in their room. They may develop phobias or have nightmares. The best way to help is to be aware of these changes and know that children always need an extra hug. They may be willing to talk at bedtime when the setting is completely relaxed. They may sometimes draw their feelings on paper.

For further information on children's grief by age and stage of development, check out the National Cancer Center Web site at www.nci.nih.gov under "Loss, Grief, and Bereavement." This site is helpful regardless of your partner's diagnosis. It also suggests books and videos you can read or watch with your children, who of course are grieving, too, and need your help and understanding.

Children and Funerals

Toni's children attended Gil's funeral, and I believe as a rule of thumb it's a good idea for kids to do so—with preparation. It's important to schedule a time to talk with them about what to expect and how to behave. Who can forget the vision of the late president John F. Kennedy's children watching his coffin pass by with Jacqueline Kennedy in widow's black? Obviously she had spoken with them in advance about what would be happening.

I've spent some time in India, where the cycle of life is a community experience. Nothing is hidden, and children are exposed to births, marriages, and deaths as part of the cycle of life. Although they may feel sad, they know death is a normal occurrence rather than something frightening. Clients who weren't allowed to attend funerals as children often wish they could have done so. You may think you are protecting youngsters by keeping them away. But doing so deprives them of an important life experience that can build character, security, and strength, instead of fear.

AFTER YOUR PARTNER IS GONE

"I always knew men died earlier than women, but it was something I read in the newspaper, just words. It happened to other people's husbands, people I didn't know. Now I understand," says Sarabeth.

Grief is indeed a process where there are no shortcuts. It can be relatively brief, or it may seem as if will continue forever. If done well, grieving can come to an end and you can continue to grow.

Although Kübler-Ross's concept of the stages of grief has become a common way to look at the process of bereavement, others exist. For example, the National Cancer Institute conceptualizes four primary stages, and in her book *Living with an Empty Chair: A Guide Through Grief,* Dr. Roberta Temes further details the process.

THE JOURNEY OF BEREAVEMENT

WHEN GRIEVING, MOST people experience variations of the following stages:

1. **Shock and numbness.** You may find it difficult to believe the death has actually occurred, and you see the world through a haze, going through the motions of life but feeling little. In her best-selling book *The Year of Magical Thinking,* Joan Didion describes her husband's fatal heart attack at the dinner table. When she arrived at the hospital with his body, a hospital worker commented, "She's a pretty cool customer." This observation captures the first stage of grief.

2. **Yearning and searching.** You long for him and feel lonely. Sometimes you turn a corner and think you've seen him, momentarily forgetting he is gone. You reach for him on the other side of the bed. You feel restless and unable to concentrate.

3. **Disorganization and despair.** You feel depressed and have trouble planning for the future. Raw feelings, such as rage, surface easily and possibly uncontrollably. Your friends and relatives may fear you're "losing it." You are not. Time has healed you enough so that you no longer need your old defenses.

4. **Reorganization.** Although life as you once knew it is gone, you are now able to focus, take on new responsibilities, and

live anew. Hope has returned, and new relationships are possible. You can embrace life.

It can take at least one year, and often much longer, to complete these stages, unless your partner died after a long-term illness during which you already did your grieving. By the time death comes, you probably feel a sense of relief along with the sadness. If grieving lasts longer than two years, seek help.

When death is sudden (and especially if it's senseless, as when he's struck by an automobile or a stray bullet), you're likely to have a more complicated adjustment to the loss. A door slams shut if an aneurysm strikes him down at his desk, or he doesn't wake up one morning because of a blood clot in his lung, or a freak accident takes him. You're left shocked, stunned, and overwhelmed. Return to normality can take a long time.

STRATEGIES FOR GRIEVING

MOURNING YOUR MATE is a very lonely place. There is no easy way to end the emotional investment of a lifetime or partnership with someone you love.

In time, you move on, because you must. However, it's normal for his loss to leave a wound that gets revisited at the most unexpected moments. Years later you may watch a movie and suddenly find yourself in tears or filled with memories. Even though you gradually rebuild your life, your history together remains part of you.

Here are some time-tested strategies to get you through the process of bereavement.

Grieve in your own way.

Grief, like so many other aspects of our complex lives, can't be reduced to an absolute definition or time line. There are so many ways people handle grief. Some do so quietly and rarely cry—or cry only privately. Others may react differently. For example, I once worked with the adult children of a mother who loudly cried and ripped her clothes at her husband's funeral. The family was embarrassed that she threw herself on the casket and made a scene. My question to the children was "How did she do afterward?" In fact, she did quite well, leading an adventurous life and traveling the world for an additional twenty years. She fully expressed her grief in her own way and was able to move on.

The family's reaction to this mother's grief is not unusual. Death often makes other people uncomfortable. The anthropologist Margaret Mead said, "When a person is born we rejoice, when they're married we jubilate, but when they die we try to pretend nothing has happened." Although death is now being talked about more openly, her words still hold true.

Speak of what has happened.

Express your thoughts and describe the details of your partner's death when you wish. Talk about your fond memories of him—how you met him, how he proposed, how he loved thick steaks. Telling positive stories helps you develop an internal scrapbook of remembrances that helps heal. Memories of a good marriage tend to help us risk entering a new relationship. And don't be afraid to laugh at his foibles. Humor is a wonderful antidote to pain. Of course, you may want to speak of how courageous he was at the end, if that is true. Talking is one way to process your grief. Choose your listeners, however, since some people can't tolerate your grief and you deserve a willing, understanding ear.

Expect intense or unusual feelings.

Give yourself permission to feel angry that he wouldn't stop smoking, fell because he took reckless risks, or that he's left you forever and you wonder how you will get along without him. You may feel guilty that you didn't spend enough time with him, or at times thought it would be easier if he died. In order to heal and move on with your life, let yourself experience your pain.

Surround yourself with those who love you, but be prepared that the first special occasion without him will always be difficult: Father's Day, Thanksgiving, Christmas, birthdays, and family events, such as your daughter's wedding.

SEVEN WAYS TO SURVIVE THIS TRANSITION

YOUR MATE'S DEATH is a major life transition surrounded by strong emotions, whether you have time to prepare for it or not. You need all the love you can garner from those who are close to you during the time he has left and after he's gone.

Here's how to help yourself (and him, when that is possible):

1. **Collaborate with your partner if you can.**

    This final period can be the ultimate collaborative effort. Your life together is coming to an end, but you can use this time to rejoice in what you've accomplished, the memories, the children (if you have a family), the relationship you've forged together. Talk about how he wants to spend the rest of his days. When the actress Candace Bergen's husband, the film director Louis Malle, learned he had nine months to live after his cancer diagnosis, he wondered how many movies he could make in that time.

    Perhaps your man wants to be surrounded by family—or to travel, if that is possible. Even if he refuses to talk about death, he can still discuss arrangements for a trip he's always wanted to take.

    You may also want to help him get closer to others and

cement good relationships. He may be ready for reconciliation with estranged friends or family members.

2. Deal with regrets.

This is also a time to discuss regrets together, which brings issues into the present and heals. Then you are open to consider forgiveness. It makes his dying easier for both of you. You can allow each other permission to say, "It doesn't matter, honey."

If you wish you had bought a bigger house, he might reply, "What difference does it make?" If he wishes he had told you he loves you more often, you can respond, "Well you can tell me now." Maybe you both regret that you didn't plan finances better. Accept the reality of the situation. And spend your last moments together with a generosity of spirit, not censure. Regrets can be painful, but if they aren't addressed at some point, they can block the way to a meaningful life ahead for you.

3. Help your partner tell his story.

History survives for the present and future generations when you record your mate's words. For example, you might:

- Tape-record his memories (and stories from others that he can listen to).
- Make videos for posterity so that your grandchildren can know him.
- Keep journals where you can write down his words (and/or others' words about him).

If he has a condition that gradually affects his faculties, such as Alzheimer's disease, try to capture his thoughts before his mental capacity completely deteriorates. Then they can be heard again and again.

4. Watch out for yourself.

"Another year of his being ill, and I'd be dead," says Sarabeth. "It was so intense and stressful. I'd come home from the hospital at night so tired. I'd walk the dog and fall into bed. After he died, I thought I'd never get my mind back. I couldn't talk. I would start a sentence and I couldn't finish it."

Sarabeth simply puts a human face on the statistics. Studies show that caregivers are at greater risk of developing serious illness after a loved one dies. Your mate's death increases your own risk of death. This is a crucial time to pay attention to your health.

Sadness is normal. There's little you can do about it except allow yourself to feel it fully, as painful as that is. If you do, in time the sadness will fade. Be aware that you are at high risk for depression now and depression is treatable. Get help when you need it. Antidepressants helped Toni and many other women in your situation get through their ordeal.

Gloria Steinem, who married for the first time at sixty-six, lost her husband three years later to lymphoma of the brain. She said in a television interview that she now knows the difference between sadness and depression. In depression, she said, nothing matters; in sadness, *everything* matters.

5. Consider a bereavement group.

Your place of worship, hospice, hospitals, the organization for his disease, or caregiver organizations can help you find bereavement groups specifically for spouses who have also lost mates. Groups may meet weekly or less often.

For example, Toni found her bereavement group very useful after Gil's death. "A lot of the people say, 'Why me?' but I don't feel that way. I don't think he did, either. I loved him, but I didn't feel he was the love of my life, as some women in the group do," she reports. "I remember feeling how strange it was for me to say I was a widow. You never think your husband will die now or that the kids won't have a father. At first, I felt I was wearing a heavy, itchy woolen overcoat that didn't fit. Suddenly, after a year, the coat became fitted cashmere—I was becoming part of who I now am." Her sons attended an eight-week bereavement group for children their age and then once-a-month meetings for a while thereafter.

Such groups can be a source of new friends as you embark on the next stage of your life. They can also help you deal with your feelings and provide the kind of comfort and support that only those who have "been there" can offer. On the other hand, some people do not find bereavement groups helpful. They don't want to listen to others' stories. This is a decision you must make for yourself.

If a group isn't your choice, you may find therapy that focuses on getting you through your grief can be useful. For some, therapy plus a group works best. In my practice, I've found that those who get stuck in the grief process don't move on as well as those who work it through.

6. Live your life.

"The worst part of bereavement is that terrible feeling of being alone," says Sarabeth. After Larry died, she stayed with her daughter in San Diego for a few months. During this time, she decided on a plan to change her life. She and Larry had been dependent on each other and didn't have many friends. Sarabeth's social circle consisted mainly of office pals. She decided she didn't want to go back to work, because it would interfere with meeting new people and getting involved in outside activities. "I'd be okay during the day. At night, in my soul, I'd still be alone," she says.

Sarabeth made a real effort to socialize. She became more active in a women's group at church that she had participated in earlier. She also joined a New Beginnings senior citizens group at church. And she started a new routine: now if she wants to see a movie or a play, she asks neighbors she's known all along to go with her. She attends local lectures, community events, and a regular yoga class, and walks long distances two days a week with a friend. "I'm out there," she says.

Sarabeth knows women who never made a new life for themselves. She didn't want that for herself. "It's strange how you can get into feeling that nobody's quite perfect enough to be the friend you want, so you don't reach out to people. But I won't do that. Having friends is much better than being fussy."

Toni had her first date a year after Gil died. She contacted an old boyfriend, and found it was wonderful to be with someone she had known in the past. Another wife, who took care of her husband for over a decade, didn't wait that long. A good man she knew approached her and said he wanted to see her when she was ready. Two weeks after her husband's death, she called the man. They had a few dinners together and enjoyed each other. Then they went to a motel one night, where after long years of abstinence, she was able to glory in her sexuality. Her husband had freed her to find happiness. He had made her promise that she wouldn't die with him and would find someone to love.

7. Be prepared for others' reactions.

Sometimes the reactions of other people can complicate your new life. Friends who have been steadfast may celebrate your quick recovery and your happiness, while others (often those who drifted away) may be unable to share your joy. Sadly, if someone has not grieved with you all along, he or she may not approve of you for achieving a new life so soon.

I remember my client Estelle, whose beloved husband's decline from Lou Gehrig's disease took a fifteen-year toll. By the time he died, she was more than ready to start a new life. One of her daughters had grieved with her and in the process even decided to go to medical school. Another daughter visited rarely while her father was sick, and denied his illness.

Soon after her husband's death, Estelle met and married a widower who was a wonderful match. The daughter who hadn't grieved wouldn't accept the remarriage, and cut off ties with her mother in a rage. This long and painful saga has yet to be resolved. Sometimes healing can take years in such situations, and the best you can do is leave the door open. You have a right to happiness.

THERE IS LIFE AFTER LOSS

A famous surgeon succumbs to lung cancer. A TV journalist dies of leukemia. A rock star loses a long battle with diabetes. Reading the obituary section of any newspaper reminds us no one is spared. Whether our partners are rich or poor, celebrities or unknowns, loss happens to us all.

In the aftermath, I have sat with people in the depths of searing pain, where all I could do was hold out hope for the future and bear witness to the validity of their experience. Yet I've seen again and again that people are enormously resilient. A remarkable number eventually recover from loss and go on to build a life. Chances are, you're a lot tougher than you realize.

Reflections

- ❧ *Help your partner die in a way that's right for both of you.*

- ❧ *Plan together in advance, if possible.*

- ❧ *Live the time left as fully as you can together.*

- ❧ *Remember, you're especially vulnerable to health problems now. Take care of yourself.*

- ❧ *Heal with hope and forgiveness. You have a future.*

16

Advice for Male Caregivers

If you're reading this chapter, your wife or partner is (or has been) ill, and you're probably in charge or playing the major supporting role. Perhaps she's been diagnosed with breast cancer or tests reveal dangerously blocked arteries. Or maybe she's suffered for years with a chronic disease like arthritis or diabetes. Whatever the diagnosis, you may feel that although you made a commitment to love her, you never signed on for *this*. You said the words "in sickness and in health," but had no idea what they could really mean. How could you? How could anyone who hasn't gone through it before? You may want to do your best to take care of her, but despite how much she means to you, somewhere deep down perhaps you doubt that you are cut out for such a role.

If you relate to any or all of the thoughts above, you have plenty of company. Over the years, I've worked with men who were thrust into taking care of an ill partner. Unprepared as they were for their new role, they found that they could commit to do the job well. Few started out as knights in shining armor.

And even those who did found themselves on a rough ride. However, those who hung in there gradually became more competent (and in some ways exceptional) at helping their mates. In the process, they often had to face buried feelings and find new ways to express their love and new approaches that made their task easier. With intention and willingness to use available resources, they came through for their partners. Each man found it is possible to make a difference for her—to be "good enough." Being "good enough" can be an extraordinary experience for you, too.

TAKING ON AN UNFAMILIAR ROLE

IT'S NOT COMMON knowledge, but four out of ten caregivers for family members today are men. Yet the whole issue of caregiving is uncharted territory for most men and usually creates ambivalent feelings. Men are often overwhelmed, frightened, conflicted, and have little idea of who to turn to for help. It is only since the 1960s, as women increasingly worked outside the home and gender roles blurred, that male caregiving became a recognized role. There were few models to draw from. The male nurses we take for granted today were rare. All of that is in the process of changing. Your partner's illness is an opportunity to grow. If you feel ill equipped and uncomfortable in your new role, it is understandable.

A contributing factor to the position you're in is your relationship to the patient. We know that the strain of caregiving is greatest when the person is your spouse. It makes sense. Marriage is an intense, all-encompassing relationship. When your wife is incapacitated, whether in the short or long term, it affects *your* life. Chances are, she is not only your lover but also your friend, the manager of the family, and the one who keeps the household (and often your social life) humming along.

Depending on her condition, her companionship may be less available than in the past. The responsibilities she handled that you always took for granted may fall to you, at least temporarily. If you feel stressed out and alone, you have good reason.

PROVIDING WHAT SHE NEEDS

HER ILLNESS RAISES other issues you probably have never coped with before. One of your key tasks is giving her what she wants and needs. If you're like many men, you may not know what that is. For example, you probably tend to think in terms of solving problems. If her medication isn't working well, your inclination is to call the doctor for a different prescription. You want to fix it. That always seems like the right thing to do. But there's more to taking care of her than solving her problems. She also needs your empathy and affection. She needs you to touch her, hold her, and talk to her. This may require you to make some changes. The jokes about women using many more words than men exist because they are generally true. By the time you've used up your allotment, she's just getting started.

Although you probably go to the bottom line, you may find she wants to talk endlessly. She may give you orders that make you bristle. Or she may expect you to read her mind and know what she wants without giving you any input. Suddenly you feel you're expected to be a psychic or a servant. How do you begin to bridge this communication gap?

On top of these challenges, you may feel confused about her response to your help. She can seem annoyed or ungrateful, or complain that the tea she requested is the wrong kind or that you don't wash the kitchen sink properly. Freud asked, "What do women want?" It is a question men have been asking ever since. Discovering what your wife wants makes your task a lot easier and allows you to be more effective for her. I describe a simple tool to help—the Husband Manual on pages 179–181. Take a look at it. The manual is a roadmap that tells women how their mates want to be taken care of. I also describe a Wife Manual that works the same way and can be useful for you. Ask your spouse to write a Wife Manual, where she lists in detail what she needs from you.

One of the things she probably needs is for you to take responsibility for unfamiliar tasks from beginning to end. If she's recovering from a hip replacement and you're making dinner, she probably wants you to figure out where the butter is located in the refrigerator instead of asking her. When you run out of sugar, she's likely to want you to replenish the supply yourself. If you don't want to do such chores and can afford it, maybe you should consider hiring a housekeeper. Remember, you've been asked to take on a demanding new role. This is no time to fly solo.

In fact, men are far more likely than women to delegate and hire outside assistance if they can. That skill can be a big advantage.

FACING UNWANTED FEELINGS

WITH SOME EXCEPTIONS, a wife's illness tends to throw otherwise strong, capable men into a tailspin. You may not know what to do, and more important, you may not know how to handle your own strong emotions. Such feelings make most guys feel vulnerable, a state they don't usually tolerate well. Denying these feelings to make them go away can work for a while. In the long run, however, ignoring your feelings usually makes life more difficult for you and everyone else who needs you. It helps to know that these deep, painful emotions aren't "wimpy"—they're perfectly normal. Virtually every man in your situation struggles with them.

Among the emotions you may feel are the following:

Helpless. You have all the responsibility and little or no control over recovery or the course of her illness. Helplessness tops the list of unwanted feelings men encounter and it can lead to feeling hopeless.

Overwhelmed. Along with your job responsibilities you now have to balance your work life with taking care of your partner. You may have always shared household (and perhaps child care) tasks. Now she's unable to do her part; *all* of it may fall on your shoulders. Helping is one thing; taking charge is another. If asked to step in and attend to your kids' needs, you may feel tense and stressed. Max, whose wife has kidney disease, told me, "I've always been a sports junkie. Now I'm Mr. Mom learning the ropes. I never thought about what clothes the girls need for school. I wish I had a set of directions telling me what to do."

Or perhaps you were looking forward to joint retirement. Now you're faced with tasks you never anticipated. "How can I begin to carve out time for myself?" you ask.

On the other hand, Scott felt threatened when his wife hired someone to come in and clean the house once a week to relieve him of the chore. "I felt it was an attack on my caregiving and on my ability to keep things going," he says. "I felt I had to do all this, and it was getting harder and harder." This attitude can lead to burnout. Although talking to others can help prevent burnout, men don't tend to share their intimate feelings with one another.

Scared and anxious. It's common to fear that (a) you won't be able to take good care of her; (b) she will die; (c) you'll have to bring the kids up all by yourself (if you have children); or (d) that you are not as invulnerable as you always assumed. If your wife or partner faces a life-threatening illness, it becomes clear that you won't live forever, either.

It's difficult to watch the woman you love in pain or in jeopardy. What if the treatment doesn't work? What if she takes a turn for the worse? What if she becomes increasingly dependent and requires more and more help and time out of your own life? Any man in your situation worries about these possibilities.

Frustrated. Patience may not be one of your virtues. If your wife's recovery is slow or there are setbacks, it may be hard to bear. If she has a chronic illness, it may frustrate you to accept that problems can't always be solved.

Sad. Every serious illness causes some kind of loss for the caregiver, whether it's loss of a sense of security and peace of mind or loss of the lifestyle you had. It's hard to accept the loss of what might have been, of hopes and dreams. You may never be able to drive cross-country again or make that trip to Tahiti together.

Angry. It's normal to rage at the disease, at the unfairness of this blow, at your wife for getting sick, at the loss of your plans for the future. Neither of you deserve this.

These are conflicting feelings, and it's likely that you prefer not to deal with them or don't know how to face them. If you've always shared your feelings with your wife, not with your buddies, you may feel lost. In this vacuum you have to pay attention to your emotions, and if you can, try to verbalize them. Difficult as it may be to open up, it's best to talk with people you trust and find safe places where you can voice concerns. This means reaching out in new ways. It's difficult to help your partner unless you can do this.

When you bottle up all those feelings, you're asking for trouble. If you don't learn how to deal with them productively, they can leak out in the form of anxiety, depression, obsessive behavior, or sleep and health problems. Your partner needs you. A stiff upper lip will get you nowhere, except perhaps sick.

Many men become so overwhelmed that they freeze up, close up, or even go away by numbing themselves with alcohol or overwork. In a short-term crisis, they pull through. In long-term debilitating illness, some marriages or long-term relationships end, with men more likely to leave than women. This is not because men are uncaring, but because they often feel frustrated and unable to face their own sense of helplessness.

There are better ways to cope—better for her, better for you, and better for your couple relationship. If you can get over resistance to seeking help, it is usually available in various forms.

BUILDING SUPPORT

OUR AMERICAN CULTURE often teaches you from childhood that asking for help isn't "macho." To be a "real man," you're supposed to be self-sufficient and take care of problems all by yourself. This attitude sets you up for trouble. It's next to impossible to take care of a sick partner, go to work, oversee the kids, and keep your home life from falling apart without assistance. Even if it's just the two of you, this is a time to turn to others for practical aid and emotional sustenance.

For example, Mike, an industrial equipment salesman in Chicago, had to cope for decades with his wife's debilitating heart disease and multiple surgeries. He frequently had to travel out of town Monday through Thursday for his job, but she often needed help. He found ways to work it out. His wife's sister and some good friends got her to the hospital when he was away. Volunteers from their church came when she was discharged.

"I stayed home when I had to and handled accounts from an office in the den. You have to give up a lot in your career unless you hire help, and that's so expensive. Most can't afford it. You work with what you've got. My church family and our relatives were very supportive," says Mike.

In general, men tend to bond over activities like sports and work. They have fewer intimate friends than women. In addition, friends often disappear when a mate is ill. They don't mean to be unavailable; they just don't know what to do. As a result, they do nothing. Many men will not pick up the phone to call and ask, "How are you managing?" On top of everything else you have to do, you may have to tell your buddies that their aid is welcome or needed (or have a family member tell them if you can't).

Participation in your religious community can be a big help, as it was for Mike. Extra social support is important, since your greatest support—your wife—may be unable to give you all you need while she's sick.

THE QUESTION OF SEX

When your wife or partner is ill, every area of life may be affected, including your sex life. For some men, it may be a relief not to have to perform. Sex may not be a priority. However, most guys do not want to give up that aspect of life. If sex is important and significant for you, it is crucial to know what your partner is thinking, whether she feels her needs are being attended to, and what your own needs are.

You may want sex because that's how you are intimate with your wife. You need physical sharing, and making love is important to your emotional well-being. In many diagnoses, however, there may be physiological changes that compromise your partner's ability to have intercourse, at least temporarily. Your own fear and stress may affect your desire and performance.

One thing to do is bring your concern out into the open and talk about it together. If that's not possible, you're still stuck with your feelings. Her current physical state may turn you off. You may feel like a married widower and have thoughts about taking your sexuality elsewhere. Many couples find it uncomfortable to discuss sex. If you're among them, this can be a time when talking with a therapist can be helpful.

It's just as important to educate yourself about sex and your wife's disease. Questions can arise for you, such as, "How will our sex life change? Will intercourse be possible? Will I hurt her?" Learn what to expect in her case, and don't assume. Too often, misunderstandings and misinformation cause confusion. Often your fears are unfounded, or there are ways to make workable adjustments. (See chapter 12 for more information on sex and serious illness.)

For example, Keith and Melanie avoided sex after Melanie's hysterectomy. Painful intercourse is often a side effect of the surgery, and both partners were afraid to try it. However, it is possible to eliminate discomfort. This couple had to learn new ways to be intimate before intercourse. They added a lot more kissing and caressing. They also visited a sex shop to investigate the latest lubricants. If you aren't comfortable with sex shops, ask your doctor for suggestions or research sex aids on the Internet.

You may feel upset if your wife has had breast reconstruction after mastectomy for breast cancer. Her breasts may feel different. It's helpful to understand that you're dealing with a new body part. Anything new and strange causes anxiety. You may also worry that you won't find your wife attractive. In his book *Breast Cancer Husband,* Marc Silver suggests that looking at a picture of a mastectomy patient can help prepare you.

For Jeff, an aeronautical engineer, the first five years of his marriage were wonderful—until his wife was diagnosed with a rare degenerative disease. As her health problems worsened, she became less and less able to respond sexually. Fatigue contributed to her lack of desire. The couple went to a sex therapist, who had some good ideas. But as the illness progressed, Jeff increasingly found himself masturbating. "I didn't have genuine desire. I craved a response from her and wasn't getting it. So much of sex is in the brain."

In a case like this, masturbation may be your way to cope. On the other hand, many men have to learn that sex is more than intercourse. It involves touching, caressing, and talking.

In the end, you have to honor your own needs, and this is a place where a caregiver support group, whose members are in similar situations, can help.

CHANGE IS POSSIBLE

MANY MEN WHO are providing care for an ill spouse think, "I can't do this." Yet the story of my former clients Morton Kondracke, the respected journalist and TV political pundit, and his wife, Milly, illustrates how one man, who was previously unsuited to take care of a sick mate, grew into the caregiving role. Milly was diagnosed with Parkinson's disease in 1988, when she was only forty-seven. Morton was a Midwesterner who was well schooled in the gut-it-out-alone and too-proud-to-need-help tradition. To the outside world, he was a well-known personality. Inside, he felt inadequate, unfulfilled, and often unable to express his love to his wife.

Mort decided that with the help of God and therapy, he would do everything he could to be with Milly until the end. He attended both individual and group therapy, where he talked about his greatest fears. He was afraid he couldn't survive without Milly and that he would lose his daughters, because Milly was the family "glue." Group members helped him deal with these concerns. They pointed out strengths he hadn't seen in himself before and suggested ways he could grow closer to his children, such as e-mailing them regularly.

As Milly's condition declined, my concern was helping them to keep their marriage alive. One of my goals was to enable them to communicate and hang on to their sense of connection. Since Mort was a writer, I suggested he write about their love story with Milly's help. For Mort, this was a way to express feelings he'd never articulated before. For Milly, who was the repository of family memories, it was a way to be involved. Even when Milly could no longer speak, they devised a sign language. She'd lift one finger for a yes and two fingers for no. Eventually the signals became eye blinks.

This story is bittersweet. The bitter part is that nothing was able to save Milly, although Mort published his best-selling book, *Saving Milly: Love, Politics, and Parkinson's Disease,* which also became a television movie. The sweet part is that Mort became a more confident, self-assured man. After Milly's death, eventually he met and married a wonderful woman. I was privileged to attend his wedding.

SIX WAYS TO DO YOUR BEST

YOU'RE ASSAULTED BY change when your partner is ill, and you may wonder how you ever wound up in this spot. But you have a job to do. Here's how to do it well as events unfold:

1. **Use your business skills to make the situation work.**

   If your wife has handled family matters in the past, the job falls to you when she's incapacitated. This is a time to delegate, a skill you're probably good at. Ask friends, mobilize family members and others to help with kids' schedules, carpooling, practices, school pick-ups, and your other new responsibilities. I know you may hate to ask for help, but her illness disrupts family and social life. It doesn't mean you love her any less if you sometimes call on substitutes to accompany her to doctors' appointments.

Turn to the Internet, as well as to her doctor, to learn all you can about her illness. If there's a voluntary organization for her disease, such as the American Cancer Society, Arthritis Foundation, or American Stroke Association, check out its Web site. Such organizations can be treasuries of information and offer (or steer you to) other kinds of help. For example, you may have to help your kids talk about their feelings and how they're coping with events around them. You have a responsibility to get direction. It's not enough just to say, "I'm paying the bills and keeping things together." Social workers can often advise you on how to navigate this new territory. There may also be counseling available for your children, if necessary.

2. Redefine what it means to be a strong man.

It takes courage and strength to be the man she needs now. Strength means increasing your ability to face your feelings so that they don't get in the way of helping her. Strength means developing empathy for her, and being there in a meaningful way for your children. Mort Kondracke did it. So did the actor Gene Wilder, who established the Gilda Radner Ovarian Cancer Detection Center after Gilda, his wife, died of the disease at age forty-two. So have many ordinary men of courage. If it is important to you, you too, can be brave.

Take a peek at the rest of this book for help. Read the chapters that seem most pertinent to your situation. You may want to try the quiz on pages 24–26 that helps caregivers identify their coping style in adversity. Although this book aims at women caregivers, it includes information and tools that can be useful for you, too.

3. Take care of you.

On average, women live more than five years longer than men. Stop kidding yourself that you're a superman. Despite all the macho messages you may hear, men are the more vulnerable sex when it comes to heart disease and cancer. If that doesn't give you enough pause, keep in mind that taking care of a sick mate takes a heavy toll.

Ask yourself, "Am I depressed?" As a caregiver, you are especially vulnerable to depression. Anger and irritability are signs of this sometimes debilitating condition. (See page 86 for a complete checklist of symptoms.) Make sleep a priority, too. Sleep deprivation contributes to depression and saps your energy.

Keep up with your golf day, poker night, or dinner with the guys. Go to the gym if you enjoy it. You have to stay mentally sound and physically healthy, or you won't be in any shape to help your wife effectively. Take your breaks, as Alec does. He went skiing several times during his wife's one-year recovery from back surgery, returning refreshed and available for her.

4. Consider therapy.

Your wife's illness puts stress on your marriage, and couples therapy is useful to open up communication between the two of you. Too often couples don't talk about the disease with each other. Invariably one person is what I call the "dragger" and the other the "draggee." When a man has to be the caregiver, he is often the draggee to therapy. Denial (or even leaving the relationship in some way) seems to him a better method of handling his fears and other emotions.

Group therapy helped my client Fred get in touch with his feelings and become a supportive coach for his wife,

Kathleen. Fred was a tax attorney who married for the first time in his fifties. Just three months later Kathleen was diagnosed with lung cancer. It was then that he came to me.

Because tasks help banish anxiety and distract the person, I suggested that Fred accompany Kathleen to doctor's appointments, take notes, and ask questions. He was good at this. Because he was surrounded by friends and willing family, he also took charge of assigning people to handle the avalanche of concerned e-mails and cards. As Fred tackled these challenges, he grew stronger and more confident, as well as more deeply in love with his wife.

So far, Kathleen has been through intensive treatment. Her prognosis is good, but there will always be uncertainty in their life. Yet Kathleen and Fred have matured as a couple. They try to appreciate every day as a precious gift.

5. Think about a support group.

Support groups are different from therapy groups, because they focus on a single disease or a single issue (as in caregiver support groups). One man whose wife had a disabling neurological disease joined the Well Spouse Association, a national nonprofit organization offering support to caregivers whose spouses are chronically ill or disabled.

He explains, "I wish I had known about the organization earlier. I couldn't talk about the pressures I felt until I joined. I went to a respite weekend, which was a revelation. People listened and didn't make excuses to get away from me. They were going through similar experiences. After a while I could attend and have fun."

Although support groups are not for everyone, they are a way of finding out what has worked for others and how to get through difficult situations. Most men tend to be more comfortable in support groups that emphasize information.

Groups can be lifesavers in situations like Alzheimer's disease, where changes in a wife's cognitive function and personality place an overwhelming burden on you.

6. **Find the right solutions for you.**

"You have to really love your wife to wait on her all these years," says Mike, the husband who had to travel for his job. "I know Type A's who wouldn't do it, but we got married for life and we're really close. She'd do anything for me, and I'd do anything for her. I knew early on she'd always have a serious heart condition."

Mike and his wife also volunteer as a couple for Mended Hearts. "You can always find people in worse shape than you are. You find out how to cope through the monthly meetings, and we always feel better after making visits to patients. You receive as much as you give," says Mike.

Another man whose wife developed dementia in her fifties refuses to put her in a nursing home. He vows to take care of her himself as long as he's alive. But not everyone feels that way. The measure of love is not necessarily based on whether you take care of your partner personally. What's important is getting her taken care of and doing the best for all of you.

Sometimes a male or female caregiver becomes attracted to someone else. Walter, a New York businessman who took care of his disabled wife for many years, found himself drawn to another woman, who also had a sick spouse. They had an intimate relationship. "I wasn't looking, but it happened. It felt so good and natural after all those years of lost intimacy. We both vowed to be there for them—and we were, until the end in both cases. But there's so much guilt. I wish it had been otherwise," he says. The couple plans to marry.

Remember, you're vulnerable to kindness and close-ness at this time. If you are attracted to someone else, a group may be able to help you sort out your feelings. For example, some men in support groups for Alzheimer's caregivers develop outside relationships, and group members have been known to support this choice.

DECIDING TO DO THE JOB WELL

IT'S PERFECTLY NORMAL to feel inadequate when your wife's illness changes your life. It isn't easy to take care of her, and you have much to learn. But I've seen men step up to the plate for the women they love. You can make the decision to be there for your wife yet honor your own needs at the same time.

Reflections

- *This difficult time is an opportunity to grow and change. Grab it.*

- *Beware of macho attitudes that undermine your effectiveness.*

- *Your instinct may be to deny how ill she is or to run. There are other, positive options.*

- *Many men have a hard time talking about feelings. That's a good reason to reach out to a support group or therapy.*

- *Remember, you can do what's right for her and take care of yourself, too.*

17

Survival Lessons

The Book of Proverbs tells us: "A woman of valor, who can find? Her price is far above rubies." You may not think these words apply to you if you are taking care of an ill mate. But I believe differently. I have seen women face catastrophes they thought they'd never survive, then find the courage to pick themselves up and go on. I know what it takes to get your mate through a major medical crisis—or an entire series of them. I've seen the stamina required day after day to help him manage a chronic illness. Although you may not see yourself as brave or heroic, I see your resilience. I know about the times you feel as if you're falling apart and want to quit, yet somehow find strength that sustains. Your value speaks for itself. I've been privileged to talk to many women who have risen to the demands thrust upon them. They tend to protest that they've done what they had to do. In fact, most have done much more.

One such woman is thirty-five-year-old Gail, who probably saved her husband's life. Gail began to see a radical personality change in her husband, a television cameraman. Always a mild-mannered man, he grew cranky, argumentative, and judgmental. His difficult behavior progressed to a point where Gail dreaded spending time with him. Sometimes she thought about leaving. In the end, two issues convinced her to stay and fight for her ten-year-old marriage: her toddler twins and nagging questions about why he had changed so much. Certain that something was terribly wrong with him—he now had alarming memory lapses as well—Gail badgered him to see a doctor. Many tests later, he was diagnosed with a rare tumor. It had to be removed within weeks or he would die.

When Gail rushed to make an appointment with the surgeon who might be able to save his life, she was told by his receptionist, "We can't see your husband until next week." Gail proceeded to scream at her, "My husband is dying and this surgeon is going to see him *now*." The receptionist squeezed in an appointment the next day. Later, when Gail needed critical test results and was told she had to wait three days for the information, she resorted to another tool in her arsenal of tactics: she cried, and got the results right away. She tailored her approach to the personality of the individual standing in the way.

This is a story with a happy ending. The delicate surgery went well, and Gail's husband was able to start easing back to work a month later. "I was relentless," she admits. "This was my twins' father, and they weren't going to grow up without him. I did what I had to do. He's alive today due to a pushy wife and good doctoring."

Not everyone's story is quite so dramatic or has such a positive outcome, of course. Some tales are more like Loretta's. At fifty-three, Loretta cares for her husband Lou, who has chronic obstructive pulmonary disease. The condition, which interferes with normal breathing, has progressed over a number of years and dramatically weakened him. Loretta must help him shower, and washes his hair.

"The worst is when he can't breathe, which happens once or twice a month. He has to concentrate on staying calm, and I can't say a word. I just have to be there. It's terrible, and all I can do is pray 'Let's get it back. Let's get it back.' It only lasts about five minutes, but it seems like an hour," she says.

When Loretta babysits for her grandchildren three days a week, Lou helps when he can. He also encourages her to go out and do things she enjoys on her own. He can't take walks with her, but Loretta is trying to persuade him to get a scooter. "We went to an inn for my birthday, and if he'd had one, he could have come with me to all the shops," she explains as her eyes light up.

Loretta sees the glass as half full, despite her narrowed life. "The disease has brought us closer. It's enabled us to spend more time together. We can't bowl, but we enjoy each other's company. We play Scrabble-type games a lot—him on one computer and me on the other. He gets to see his grandchildren all the time. Life doesn't end. You do what you *can* do."

Sandy, a fifty-eight-year-old Pasadena homemaker, was less fortunate. Her husband's dementia robbed her of the man she adored. He gradually deteriorated to a point where he couldn't be left alone for even five minutes. Despite pleas from her doctor, and days when she felt like she couldn't go on, Sandy refused to put her husband in a nursing home and hired help instead. He was able to die at home as he would have wished.

"I was married to him for twenty-eight years, and I don't think you leave a sinking ship," she says. "I like to think that he'd do the same thing for me."

Sandy has no regrets, and today she has a new relationship with a widower in her neighborhood. "I don't think I could be in this relationship or be the person I am if I hadn't done what I did. I feel very lucky to have met someone who is gentle and kind and has the same likes and dislikes I do. I loved my husband very much, but after what I've been through, this man is the perfect one for me. We're getting married in a few months. There *is* life after death."

Some of us might have chosen a different path from Sandy's. Can there be anything lonelier or more painful than living with someone who is an empty shell? But each and every one of us is different; our significant relationships are different. We do our best and hope it is good enough.

SIX WAYS YOUR PARTNER'S ILLNESS MAY HAVE CHANGED YOU

SANDY, LORETTA, AND Gail consider themselves quite ordinary—and in many ways they are. Yet they have been through a crucible that has forged them into stronger people. Your partner's illness has undoubtedly tested you and changed you in a number of ways:

1. **You may have become proactive.**

   Chances are, you've learned new skills, which may include speaking up to doctors and support staffs as Gail did, or asking in the ambulance for the best emergency room to handle a heart attack victim. You may know the drill when he gets another blood clot in his leg. Or you may have learned to stand up to your mate and call 911 over his protests when your gut tells you it's necessary.

   Maybe you can relate to another wife who fought to make her apartment building wheelchair-accessible for her husband. When the landlord refused, she called her city's Commission on Human Rights—and won.

   Some people become proactive in other ways. They may start their own support groups when appropriate ones aren't available in their communities—or even start their own organizations. For instance, Suzanne Mintz is president and cofounder of the National Family Caregivers Association, and Maggie Strong, author of *Mainstay,* founded the Well Spouse Association.

You may have had other experiences you never anticipated that have made you stronger. As one woman explains, "I don't get hysterical anymore when he has a setback. I'm used to little bumps in the road. They are nothing."

2. You may have learned to set limits.

There's a difference between selfless love and selfdestruction. It's selfless to encourage your husband's desire to connect with his family when you can't abide them. It's self-destructive to work yourself into exhaustion being his nurse 24/7 because you're too proud to ask for (or look for) help, or have a distorted sense of duty.

Every caregiver struggles with balancing compassionate care and self-care. A big question at this time is, "Can you live a life even if it's harder than you expected?" The answer is likelier to be yes if you take the time you need for yourself.

You may also have learned to set boundaries with other people and say no. One wife sent her visiting mother-in-law home. The woman's bossiness gave her panic attacks as her husband recovered from life-threatening surgery. If other people are debilitating you, you have to do what you must to function.

3. You may have learned to become more vulnerable.

Many women cry in a corner, but you may now let tears come as they may. You may have taken a risk and reached out. A committed partner recalls how angry she felt that she didn't get enough support when her partner injured his back and faced months of rehabilitation.

People had the impression that she was a rock capable of dealing with any obstacle, but at the same time she fumed at them for failing to offer help. She felt she shouldn't have to ask for it.

"It was my own stupidity and stubbornness. My pride wouldn't let me ask for help, and people told me they didn't know I needed anything," she says.

4. You may have learned more about yourself.

You may have figured out the main stress points between you and your mate and discovered that the problem is sometimes you, not just him. Helplessness is a painful cross to bear, but it isn't always negative. It can make you humble. For example, a client of mine, a very successful CEO, was not at her best in a caregiving role. An aggressive person who fought her way to the top of the company ladder, she handled her husband's hip replacement the same way she handled business. She took charge, issued orders, and told him (and everyone else) what he needed. Her actions alienated both him and the hospital staff.

Finally, a friend pointed out that her husband seemed to wither under her approach. She had to learn to listen rather than tell. Wise and loving woman that she is, she was able to avoid becoming defensive and to realize that her controlling behavior had to change. A take-charge attitude was useful at times and made her feel better, but it hurt him.

You may have discovered you can be more flexible and tolerate ambivalence—a world of gray. Long-term illness particularly evokes many competing emotions. Feelings of desperation can go hand in hand with hope, and love with hate. It's difficult to accept these contradictions. When you do, it's easier to live with the reality of the situation and recognize the many facets of yourself. You are in fact a tapestry, which makes you wiser and more human.

5. You may have struggled to make a moral or pragmatic decision.

There are times when commitment is the only thing that pulls you through. You feel a vow is a vow. Or you stay for economic reasons or for the sake of the family. I think of Erica, who has two young daughters. Her husband, an actor, was diagnosed with rapidly progressing multiple sclerosis when he was thirty-two. The illness has affected him psychologically, causing him to go on buying binges and run up a huge debt. Right now, spending is the way he handles his fear of being immobilized in a few years. She's had to assume the unwanted role of money manager to protect the family's economic stability.

This was a troubled marriage before he got sick. He was a dreamer, disinterested in practicalities like financial security, and now Erica often feels she and the children would have a better life without him. She fears he will bankrupt them. But so far, commitment and the children keep her hanging in.

"Doing the right thing doesn't always end in happiness," says a character in the novel *Snow,* by the Nobel Prize winner Orhan Pamuk. That's true for Erica.

6. You may have started on the path toward transformational love.

"My heart never broke for him before he got sick. I never realized how much I could miss him until he was on a respirator and we couldn't communicate. I didn't truly understand what a partnership is until I didn't have it. I couldn't ask, 'What do you think we should do about—? What's your take on—?' I appreciated him so much when they finally weaned him off the machine and he was able to talk," says a wife.

Charlotte learned what a good marriage she had. She told me:

I always thought our marriage was solid, but dealing with my husband's cancer together made it stronger. We connected, communicated, and supported each other. All the small stuff we had always been so concerned about, like what kind of car we should buy, seemed so trivial. Only important issues remained—saving his life and nurturing our relationship. I read an article on love that said first you have attraction, then a comfort level, and eventually partnership. We have that. We work as a team. We still disagree at times, but we can argue and still care for each other so much better than before his illness.

When we'd been married six or seven years, some of our friends started getting divorced. He came home one night and said, "Are we okay?" We were. We still ask ourselves that question occasionally. After thirty years, the answer is yes. He's my partner, and I'll do anything to save him.

ADJUSTING TO THE NEW NORMAL

AT SOME POINT—whether it's after treatment is completed, after he recovers from surgery, or as you manage a chronic disease—your life finds its own normal setting. The term "the new normal" has been coined to describe this phase of life, which didn't exist years ago. People got sick. Then they got better or they died. That is no longer the case. For example, there are over ten million cancer survivors today. If your mate is a survivor, you live your life as normally as you can, but what is normal has changed. There is always the underlying threat of a recurrence or other problems.

For one couple, the new normal is acceptance that he tires easily long after his successful bone marrow transplant. "We used to enjoy working together outside in the garden and doing house projects, but now we pay people to do it. We pace our social life, because he's too exhausted to go out two nights in a row. A few times a year he crawls into bed for a few days. But most people don't go back to work after this, and he did, so we're lucky," says this wife.

Part of the new normal may be changes in living arrangements that can make life easier. In some cases you may decide it's best to move to a retirement community or closer to your children. One husband is a stroke survivor who was left with poor balance and a weakness on one side. His mental capacity is not what it used to be. "Last week he ordered twenty-two bags of sugar-free candy, because it included free shipping. But he is able to do the laundry and he cooks. We go to wheelchair-accessible movies and restaurants," says his wife, Stella.

They live in a townhouse, where Stella had to convert the downstairs living room into his bedroom for a year. She keeps a walker on each floor and has made kitchen cabinets accessible for him.

You may face other issues, such as structural changes at home. Can his wheelchair get through the bathroom door? If money is tight, you may not want to redo the bathroom. Yet one partner says replacing the bathtub with a spacious shower with grab bars is the best money she ever spent. What seems like an extravagance can actually be an investment in quality of life. Emergency nightlights can help prevent a fall. This may seem like a minor detail, but it could save his life. Falls are the leading cause of injury and injury deaths for older adults.

FINDING A BALANCE

WHEN YOU'RE IN a crisis mode and rushing to the hospital or to worrisome tests and doctor's appointments, you may have to put some activities on hold to maintain your equilibrium. Perhaps you're a member of certain committees, the PTA, your professional or business organization, a knitting group. You probably get lots of satisfaction from these commitments. For a period of time, however, life as you know it may not be the same . You may have to take a hiatus until home life calms down. Only you can decide whether continuing some of your activities will support or drain you. You may wish to keep the ones you truly look forward to—maybe your online group that discusses Jane Austen, or your exercise class—and drop the others for now.

I know long-term caregivers who find ways to be realistic and have a life. This can mean many things. Sometimes living fully in the new normal means seeking closer relationships with other women. Women need companionship, to sit and talk with one another, more than men do. In fact, recent studies show that female bonding actually produces the hormone oxytocin, which helps women live longer.

A client of mine has made a conscious effort to talk with her neighbors. They've always been there, but now she takes the time to stop and chat, and trades information with one neighbor, who also has a sick husband. She gave my client a sample of a product that speeds healing of bedsores. The neighbor mentioned an antidepressant that boosted her mate's appetite and helped him gain weight. "I'll check it out with the doctor. Maybe it will work for my husband, too," my client replied. She appreciates the tips along with the sense of community.

GET CONSISTENCY INTO YOUR LIFE AGAIN

TRY TO RECOGNIZE your own need for stability and nurturance, especially if you're in a long-haul situation. Structure is your friend, and a Wednesday drawing class, a bridge club, or a weekly golf or tennis game helps ease anxiety. Make a list of activities that make you feel good and work for you, whether it's reading, seeing friends, signing up for a local chorus, or attending events that draw you out of yourself, such as theater and sports.

The Value of Volunteering

Satisfying volunteer activities are in a category all their own. Helping others makes you feel better, and it's also an opportunity to gain new skills (sometimes marketable skills), meet new people, and enlarge your social circle. For my coauthor, Florence, involvement in something totally different does the trick. She volunteers one afternoon a week at a telephone hotline run by a nonprofit agency. She says,

> *It sounds crazy. My husband is in the hospital for a month, and I feel so happy when I go to my gig on Thursday afternoons, where I handle calls for everything from domestic violence to suicide to people who are just plain lonely and need someone to talk to. Listening to other people's problems is therapy for me. My husband's health problems are largely out of my control, but here I can frequently make a difference for people. A bonus for me is another volunteer who works the same shift I do. Her husband is a cancer survivor, and we've become good friends. Talking to her has helped me a lot.*

Florence's hotline choice may not appeal to you, but there exist many other opportunities for volunteering. Volunteer work that has meaning for you adds a whole new dimension to your life.

Maintain Connections and Share Interests

Resilient people maintain connections and share interests with people outside of their home, yet many caregivers complain that isolation is a major source of stress. Don't let yourself fall into that trap.

One of my clients just saw an exhilarating photography exhibit at the art museum with an old college roommate and had lunch with her in the cafeteria. This was her third attempt to get together with her friend, but she made it. "I had to cancel two other dates, because my husband had medical emergencies. But I wouldn't let this one go. I must feed my soul, have some pleasure, and see my pals. I feel alive for the first time in a long while," she told me.

Another woman plans at least one trip a year with her sister. She spends a week "doing nothing" far away from home. The vacation makes it possible for her to return to her husband, who is largely housebound. If you don't put positives in your life to balance the negatives, it's as if you're forcing yourself to walk with a limp.

Sometimes new contacts bring unexpected pleasure. For a long time, her sister regaled Janet with stories about the Red Hat Society, a nationwide organization for women over fifty. "She loved it and had such a good time with the women she met there. I decided to check out the society's Web site and found a chapter in my state," Janet says. "It's a wonderful group of women, and we've become very close friends. We attend meetings, go on trips together, and I never would have met them if I hadn't joined the Red Hats."

Connect Even When You're Homebound

There are ways to connect with people even if you're stuck in the house. Amanda's husband is good company, and she has outlets in knitting, crocheting, and other crafts. "I never get cabin fever," she says, and has even met a friend on the Internet through a shared interest in quilting. Another client of mine met Internet friends through her passion for scrapbooking.

Over the long term, the Internet can help you break through isolation and connect you with others who share similar experiences.

Look for Role Models

DANA REEVE, WIDOW of the actor Christopher Reeve (who herself died of lung cancer in 2006), said she never thought, "This is not what I bargained for. I want out," because they had a life together, despite his profound disability. She took care of him at first, then gradually resumed her acting career, as well as wearing other hats.

People like Dana Reeve have become role models because they choose to become public and proactive. The television journalist Meredith Vieira is another woman who inspires with her ability to rise above catastrophe. She lives a life, raises three children (plus pets), and is there for her husband who is legally blind as a result of multiple sclerosis and has other health problems.

You can learn from other women, even if their lives are different from yours and they have money or other resources not available to you. Position in life does not eliminate personal struggle. You don't have to be famous to give your pain meaning.

Role models may be all around you if you pay attention: your friend's mother who has become a community leader, or the woman in the elevator who travels with her disabled husband. Can you set goals for yourself and make the time to achieve them?

A wife who has cared for her husband for years went back to school for a new career. She plans to become an empowerment coach. A career gives her peace of mind because her greatest anxiety is being a burden on her kids. Perhaps there's a goal you can consider.

MOVING ON

YOU MAY BE taking care of your partner on a temporary basis, with hope for a relatively normal life at the end of a monthlong (or longer) siege. Neither of you will ever be the same after all you've been through. But at least there is light at the end of tunnel.

Or the outcome of your mate's condition may still be uncertain. Cure may or may not be possible. He may or may not come back from his ordeal able to have a good quality of life (or any life at all).

Or the road ahead may be all too clear—more of the same in a chronic condition, or a worsening situation. This may go on for many years or even decades. The caregiving experience can forge character, strength, and compassion. But I've never met a woman who wouldn't exchange those gains for a magic wand to make her partner well. Yet there *are* rewards for what you do. "It isn't fun, but it beats being alone. At least I have the man I love" is the way one wife sums it up. You can get through this. You always do.

Back in 458 BCE, the Greek tragedian Aeschylus wrote, "Wisdom comes alone through suffering." That's still true, although the scars may not show.

Like many courageous caregivers throughout this book, you may be an ordinary woman in extraordinary circumstances. Life may have swept away your safety net and assaulted you with change. Remember all that you've accomplished and be kind to yourself. With help, you can do your best for you and your partner. Your way is good enough.

Postscript

Florence Isaacs's husband, Harvey Isaacs, had been ill several times since his mid-forties, although he always came back and was able to return to work as an attorney, and to embrace life. Sadly, a month before the completion of this book, his last illness had a different ending. He died unexpectedly on October 16, 2006.

Resources

DISEASE-RELATED ORGANIZATIONS

Alzheimer's Association
225 N. Michigan Avenue, 17th floor
Chicago, IL 60601-7633
800-272-3900
www.alz.org
info@alz.org

American Autoimmune Related Diseases Association
22100 Gratiot Avenue
East Detroit, MI 48021
800-598-4668
586-776-3900
www.aarda.org
aarda@aol.com

American Cancer Society
6525 N. Meridian, Suite 110
Oklahoma City, OK 73116
800-ACS-2345
www.cancer.org

American Diabetes Association
1701 North Beauregard Street
Alexandria, VA 22311
800-DIABETES (800-342-2383)
www.diabetes.org
AskADA@diabetes.org

American Heart Association
7272 Greenville Avenue
Dallas, TX 75231
800-AHA-USA-1 (800-242-8721)
www.amhrt.org

American Liver Foundation
75 Maiden Lane, Suite 603
New York, NY 10038
800-465-4837
888-443-7872
212-668-1000
www.liverfoundation.org
info@liverfoundation.org

American Lung Association
61 Broadway, 6th floor
New York, NY 10006
800-LUNGUSA (800-586-4872)
212-315-8700
www.lungusa.org

American Stroke Association
7272 Greenville Avenue
Dallas, TX 75231
888-4-STROKE (888-478-7653)
www.strokeassociation.org

Amyotrophic Lateral Sclerosis Association
   (Lou Gehrig's disease)
27001 Agoura Road, Suite 150
Calabasas Hills, CA 91301-5104
800-782-4747
818-800-9007
www.alsa.org

Arthritis Foundation
P.O. Box 7669
Atlanta, GA 30357-0669
800-568-4045
404-872-7100
www.arthritis.org

CancerCare
275 Seventh Avenue, 22nd floor
New York, NY 10001
800-813-HOPE (800-813-4673)
www.cancercare.org
info@cancercare.org

Christopher and Dana Reeve Paralysis Resource Center
636 Morris Turnpike, Suite 3A
Short Hills, NJ 07078
800-539-7309
www.paralysis.org

Crohn's & Colitis Foundation of America
386 Park Avenue South, 17th floor
New York, NY 10016
800-932-2423
www.ccfa.org

Huntington's Disease Society of America
505 Eighth Avenue, Suite 902
New York, NY 10018
800-345-HDSA (800-345-4372)
212-242-1968
www.hdsa.org
hdsainfo@hdsa.org

The Leukemia & Lymphoma Society
1311 Mamaroneck Avenue
White Plains, NY 10605
800-955-4572
914-949-5213
www.leukemialymphoma.org

The Mended Hearts, Inc.
7272 Greenville Avenue
Dallas, TX 75231-4596
888-HEART99 (888-432-7899)
214-360-6149
www.mendedhearts.org
info@mendedhearts.org

Myasthenia Gravis Foundation
   of America, Inc.
1821 University Avenue West, Suite S256
St. Paul, MN 55104
800-541-5454
651-917-6256
www.myasthenia.org
mgfa@myasthenia.org

National Kidney Foundation
30 East 33rd Street
New York, NY 10016
800-622-9010
212-889-2210
www.kidney.org

National Multiple Sclerosis Society
733 Third Avenue
New York, NY 10017
800-FIGHT-MS (800-344-4867)
www.nationalmssociety.org

National Organization for Rare Disorders
55 Kenosia Avenue
P.O. Box 1968
Danbury, CT 06813-1968
800-999-6673 (voice mail only)
203-744-0100
www.rarediseases.org
orphan@rarediseases.org

National Parkinson Foundation
1501 NW 9th Avenue / Bob Hope Road
Miami, FL 33136-1494
800-327-4545
305-243-6666
www.parkinson.org
contact@parkinson.org

United Ostomy Association of America, Inc.
P.O. Box 66
Fairview, TN 37062–0066
800-826-0826
www.uoaa.org
info@uoaa.org

CAREGIVER ORGANIZATIONS

Family Caregiver Alliance
180 Montgomery Street, Suite 1100
San Francisco, CA 94104
800-445-8106
415-434-3388
www.caregiver.org
info@caregiver.org

National Alliance for Caregiving
4720 Montgomery Lane, 5th floor
Bethesda, MD 20814
301-718-8444
www.caregiving.org
info@caregiving.org

National Family Caregivers Association
10400 Connecticut Avenue, Suite 500
Kensington, MD 20895-3944
800-896-3650
301-942-6430
www.nfcacares.org
info@thefamilycaregiver.org

Well Spouse Association
63 West Main Street, Suite H
Freehold, NJ 07728
800-838-0879
732-577-8899
www.wellspouse.org
info@wellspouse.org

HOSPICE ORGANIZATIONS

National Association for Home Care and Hospice
228 Seventh Street, SE
Washington, DC 20003
202-547-7424
www.nahc.org

National Hospice and Palliative Care Organization
1700 Diagonal Road, Suite 625
Alexandria, VA 22314
800-658-8898
703-837-1500
www.nhpco.org
info@nhpco.org

HEALTH AGENCIES

Centers for Disease Control and Prevention (CDC)
1600 Clifton Road
Atlanta, GA 30333
800-311-3435
404-639-3534
www.cdc.gov
info@cdc.gov

National Institutes of Health (NIH)
9000 Rockville Pike
Bethesda, MD 20892
301-496-4000
www.nih.gov
NIHinfo@od.nih.gov

National Cancer Institute (NCI)
NCI Public Inquiries Office
6116 Executive Boulevard, Room 3036A
Bethesda, MD 20892-8322
800-4-CANCER (800-422-6237)
www.cancer.gov
cancergovstaff@mail.nih.gov

National Center for Complementary and
   Alternative Medicine (NCCAM) (NIH)
9000 Rockville Pike
Bethesda, MD 20892
888-644-6226
www.nccam.nih.gov
info@nccam.nih.gov

National Heart, Lung, and Blood Institute
National Institutes of Health
NHLBI Health Information Center
Attention: Web Site
P.O. Box 30105
Bethesda, MD 20824-0105
301-592-8573
www.nhlbi.nih.gov

National Institute of Mental Health
Public Information and Communications Branch
6001 Executive Blvd., Room 8184, MSC 9663
Bethesda, MD 20892-9663
800-421-4211
www.nimh.nih.gov
nimhinfo@nih.gov

Office of Cancer Complementary and Alternative Medicine
(OCCAM)
National Cancer Institute, NIH
6116 Executive Boulevard, Suite 609, MSC 8339
Bethesda, MD 20892
888-644-6226
www.cancer.gov/cam/

OTHER HELPFUL RESOURCES

AARP
601 E Street, NW
Washington, DC 20049
800-OUR-AARP (888-687-2277)
www.aarp.org/life/caregiving

Eldercare Locator
1730 Rhode Island Avenue, NW, Suite 1200
Washington, D.C. 20036
800-677-1116
www.eldercare.gov
eldercarelocator@spherix.com

Medicare
U.S. Department of Health and Human Services
Centers for Medicare and Medicaid Services
7500 Security Blvd.
Baltimore, MD 21244-1850
800-MEDICARE (800-633-4227)
www.medicare.gov

National Organization for Empowering Caregivers
425 W. 23rd Street, Suite 9B
New York, N.Y. 10011
212-807-1204
www.care-givers.com
info@care-givers.com

Rosalynn Carter Institute for Caregiving
800 GSW Drive
Georgia Southwestern State University
Americus, GA 31709-4379
229-928-1234
www.rosalynncarter.org
rci@canes.gsw.edu

U.S. Social Security Administration
Office of Public Inquiry
Windsor Park Building
6401 Security Boulevard
Baltimore, MD 21235
800-772-1213
www.ssa.gov

Acknowledgments

My personal mantra is "Life is too hard to do alone—Reach out!" This statement's truth was constantly evident during the creation of this book. I was sustained through the months of writing and editing and rewriting by the help of those around me. Linda Konner, my agent, saw the need for this book before I did. Kathryn McHugh's support and thoughtful editing made it a better read. Skye MacBroom and Jim DeMicco of Skye Communication added flavor and a touch of spice. Dr. Mary Liston Liepold, always a steadfast friend, did double duty as compassionate critic. Jennifer Cohen, creative assistant extraordinaire, patiently picked up my life's missing pieces.

To my coauthor Florence, our differences of opinion served for a richer, more comprehensive book. Your courage and strength in dealing with the illness of your husband, Harvey, serves as a reminder that while I was writing this book, you were living it.

To my husband, Isaac, I thank you for your constant loving presence, your patient listening, and when I got too serious, your ability to make me laugh. You remained my caregiver when I needed it most and taught me a deeper dimension of love.

This book also owes its existence to my many clients who have always educated and often healed me. Most of all, with deepest respect, I acknowledge you, the caregiver. It is for you that this book has been written.

—Dorree Lynn, PhD

THE SUPPORT OF Dr. Fredrick Rapoport, a physician who never forgets his humanity or the patient's dignity, helped carry me through this project. I will always be in your debt. During this time I was also blessed with the counsel of Dr. Marvin Dorph. You were (and are) always there.

For their valuable insights, I also thank clinical psychologist Korey Hood, PhD, of the Joslin Clinic; Fr. J. Rooney, Chaplain, Pastoral Care, St. Vincent's Hospital–Manhattan; and Richard Harra, Director of Online Services, CancerCare. To the many valiant caregivers I interviewed who contributed their experiences and wisdom, you know who you are. I'll always remember you.

—Florence Isaacs

Bibliography

Allison, Jay, and Dan Gediman, eds. *This I Believe.* New York: Henry Holt and Company, 2006.

American Insomnia Association. www.americaninsomnia association.org.

Armstrong, Pamela. *Surviving Healthcare.* Concord, CA: Chestnut Ridge Books, 2004.

Berk, Lee. "The Laughter-Immune Connection: New Discoveries." *Humor and Health Journal*, vol. 5, no. 5, 1996.

Burls, Ambra, and Woody Caan. "Human health and nature conservation." *British Medical Journal*, 2005. Vol 331, p 1221–22.

Centers for Disease Control and Prevention. Morbidity and Mortality Weekly Report. November 16, 2006.

Christakis, Nicholas A., and Paul D. Allison. "Mortality after the Hospitalization of a Spouse." *New England Journal of Medicine*, 2006; 354: 719–30.

Cohen, Richard M. *Blindsided: Lifting a Life Above Illness: A Reluctant Memoir.* New York: HarperCollins, 2005.

Cousins, Norman. *Anatomy of an Illness as Perceived by the Patient.* New York: W. W. Norton & Co., 2005 (Reprint edition).

Didion, Joan. *The Year of Magical Thinking.* New York: Knopf, 2005.

Glaser, Jennifer. "Mortality Can Be a Powerful Aphrodisiac." *New York Times*, August 13, 2006.

Jerome, Jim. "No More Tears." *AARP The Magazine*, July & August 2005.

Kiecolt-Glaser, Janice K., et al. "Hostile Marital Interactions, Proinflammatory Cytokine Production, and Wound Healing." *Archives of General Psychiatry*, 2005; 62:1377–84.

Kondracke, Morton. *Saving Milly: Love, Politics, and Parkinson's Disease.* New York: Ballantine Books, 2002.

Kornblum, Janet. "Caregivers' Health in 'downward spiral.'" *USA Today*, September 25, 2006.

Kübler-Ross, Elisabeth. *On Death and Dying*. New York: Scribner, 1997.

Lublin, Joann S. "No One to Turn To." *Wall Street Journal*, October 9, 2006.

McCue, Kathleen, with Ron Bonn. *How to Help Children Through a Parent's Serious Illness*. New York: St. Martin's Griffin, 1996.

Mead, Margaret. *Male and Female*. New York: HarperCollins, 2001. (Originally published by William Morrow, 1949).

Mintz, Suzanne Geffen. *Love, Honor, & Value*. Herndon, VA: Capital Books, 2002.

Pamuk, Orhan. *Snow*. New York: Vintage Reprint Edition, 2005.

Peck, M. Scott. *The Different Drum: Community Making and Peace*. New York: Touchstone, 1998 (Reprint edition).

Prescott, Lawrence M. "Men with low PSA may not need annual screening." *Urology Times*, July 2002.

Richtel, Matt. "Past Divorce, Compassion at the End." *New York Times*, May 19, 2005.

Rolland, John S. *Families, Illness, & Disability*. New York. Basic Books, 1994.

Rosenthal, Saul M. *The New Sex Over 40*. New York: Tarcher, 1999.

Short, Pamela Farley, et al. "Employment Pathways in a Large Cohort of Adult Cancer Survivors." *Cancer*, March 15, 2005; 103: 1292–1301.

Silver, Marc. *Breast Cancer Husband: How to Help Your Wife (and Yourself) through Diagnosis, Treatment, and Beyond*. Emmaus, PA: Rodale, 2004.

Smyth, Joshua M., et al. "Brief Writing Exercises Can Reduce Symptoms in Patients with Chronic Illness." *Journal of the American Medical Association*, 1999; 281: 1304–09.

Strong, Maggie. *Mainstay: For the Well Spouse of the Chronically Ill*. Cambridge, MA: Bradford Books, 1997.

Taylor, S. E., et al. "Biobehavioral Response to Stress in Females: Tend and Befriend, Not Fight or Flight." *Psychological Review*, July 2000; 107 (3): 411–29.

Temes, Roberta. *Living with an Empty Chair*. Far Hills, NJ: New Horizon Press, 1992.

Stanford University School of Medicine. http://www.mednews .stanford.edu/releases. "Antidepressants Lessen Risk of of Heart Attack, Stanford Researcher Says." July 4, 2005.

Trief, Paula M., et al. "The Marital Relationship and Psychosocial Adaptation and Glycemic Control of Individuals with Diabetes." *Diabetes Care*, 2001; 24 (8): 1384–89.

Trief, Paula M., et al. "The Relationship Between Marital Quality and Adherence to the Diabetes Care Regimen." *Annals of Behavioral Medicine*, 2004; 27 (3): 148–54.

Wexler, David B. *When Good Men Behave Badly: Change Your Behavior, Change Your Relationship*. Oakland, CA: New Harbinger, 2004.

Index

social life, 176–177, 183–184, 285, 297, 298
    after spouse's death, 269–270
Social Security, 148, 290
social worker, 126
spirituality, 35, 90
    and end of life, 257–258
    role of, 240–243
ssa.gov (Social Security website), 148
Steinem, Gloria, 268
stoicism, 229–230
stress, 10–11
StrokeAssociation.org (website), 106
strokes
    and disability, 143, 207
    recovery from, 141
    symptoms of, 115
Strong, Maggie, *Mainstay*, 293
support
    asking for help, 40–41, 51
    community, 5–6, 39, 45–46
    delegating responsibilities, 43–44, 51–52
    employee assistance programs, 153
    from family, 42–44, 54, 64, 71, 71–72, 154
    from friends, 44–46, 53–54, 64, 154, 173
    importance of, 39–40
    lists, of possible sources, 55–56
    for male caregivers, 279–280
    professional help. *see* counseling
    resistance to, 244
support groups, 46–51
    bereavement, 268–269
    for caregivers, 154, 207
    for children, 73
    evaluating, 49–51, 52–53
    finding, 49–51
    for male caregivers, 286–287
    online, 47–48, 50
    for patients, 97–98, 152
    visiting, 48
surgery, recovery time, 130–131
Surviving Healthcare (Armstrong), 107

Tai Chi, 88
Tan, Stanley, 193
Tantric sex, 208
technology, medical, 128
teenagers, 62–63, 64–65, 66, 71
Temes, Roberta, *Living with an Empty Chair*, 263
terminal illness, 13, 253–254. *see also* death
thinker coping style, 27–28, 179–180

This I Believe (Lantry), 175
This I Believe (TV series), 240
time management, 5, 153–154, 298
training, caregiver, 23, 35
transformational love, 159–161, 295–296
    and anger, 222
    and intimacy, 171–172, 177–178
    and sexuality, 197
    steps to, 171–175
traveling, 191–192
treatment, noncompliance with, 94–96
Type A personality, 84

United Ostomy Association, 308
University of Pennsylvania, 10
unmarried partners, 137–138, 151
U.S. News and World Report, 134
U.S. Social Security Administration Office of Public Inquiry, 290

Viagra, 201, 203
Vieira, Meredith, 85, 301
volunteering, 299–300
vulnerability, patient, 83–84

Wall Street Journal, 155
websites, 106–109
    caregiver training, 35
    clinical trials, 108
    end of life, 257, 261
    financial issues, 148
    information, disease, 106–109, 113, 284
    pornographic, 202
    sexual issues, 207
    support, 39
Well Spouse Association, 49, 51, 293, 309
Wexler, David B., *When Good Men Behave Badly*, 83
what if syndrome, 216–217
When Good Men Behave Badly (Wexler), 83
Wife Manual, 182–183, 276
Wilder, Gene, 284
work. *see* employment
working women. *see* employment, caregiver
worry, 236–237. *see also* anxiety; fear

Year of Magical Thinking, The (Didion), 263
yoga, 88, 242, 247